To Mary, Peggy, Helen and Penny

He that shortens the road to knowledge
lengthens life.
  Lacon, Charles Caleb Colton (1780–1832)

To Mary, Peggy, Helen and Penny

Ostlere & Bryce-Smith's Anaesthetics for Medical Students

Thomas B. Boulton

MA, MB, BChir, FDSRCS, FFARCS DA

Consultant Anaesthetist, Nuffield Department of Anaesthetics,
Oxford and the Royal Berkshire Hospital, Reading;
Clinical Lecturer, University of Oxford

Colin E. Blogg

MB, BS, FFARCS, DObst RCOG

Consultant Anaesthetist, Nuffield Department of Anaesthetics,
Radcliffe Infirmary, Oxford.
Clinical Lecturer, University of Oxford.

With a Foreword by
The late

C. Langton Hewer

MB, BS, MRCP, FFARCS, DA

Consulting Anaesthetist, St. Bartholomew's Hospital, London.

TENTH EDITION

CHURCHILL LIVINGSTONE
EDINBURGH, LONDON, MELBOURNE AND NEW YORK 1989

CHURCHILL LIVINGSTONE
Medical Division of Longman Group UK Limited

Distributed in the United States of America by Churchill Livingstone Inc., 1560
Broadway, New York, N.Y. 10036, and by associated companies, branches and
representatives throughout the world.

First Edition 1949	Fifth Edition 1963	Eight Edition 1976
Second Edition 1951	Sixth Edition 1966	Ninth Edition 1980
Third Edition 1956	Seventh Edition 1972	Tenth Edition 1989
Fourth Edition 1960		

ISBN 0-443-02821-4

British Library Cataloguing in Publication Data
Ostlere, Gordon, *1921*
    Ostlere & Bryce-Smith's Anaesthetics for medical students. — 10th ed.
    1. Medicine. Anaesthesia
    I. Title   II. Bryce-Smith, Roger   III. Boulton, Thomas B.
    617'.96

Library of Congress Cataloging in Publication Data
Ostlere, Gordon.
    [Anaesthetics for medical students]
    Ostlere & Bryce-Smith's anaesthetics for medical students. — 10th
    ed. / Thomas B. Boulton, Colin E. Blogg; with a foreword by C.
    Langton Hewer.
        p.   cm.
    Rev. ed. of: Anaesthetics for medical students / Gordon Ostlere,
    Roger Bryce-Smith. 9th ed. 1980
    Bibliography: p.
    ISBN (invalid) 04430282214
    1. Anesthesia. 2. Anesthetics. [1. Anesthesia.] I. Boulton,
    T. B. II. Blogg, Colin E. III. Title. IV. Title: Anaesthetics for
    medical students. V. Title: Ostlere and Bryce-Smith's anaesthetics
    for medical students.
        [DNLM: WO 200 085a]   RD81.08 1989   617'.96 — dc19

Produced by Longman Singapore Publishers (Pte) Ltd.
Printed in Singapore.

Extract from the Foreword to The First Edition

There are in existence a large number of textbooks on anaesthesia, some of great merit, but none really caters for the needs of the undergraduate anaesthetic clerk.

This unfortunate individual is in process of acquiring and retaining (until his final examinations) a huge assortment of facts and theories, and the short time that he can spare for anaesthesia must be essentially practical.

Dr Ostlere does not fall into the common error of attempting to explain the scientific reasons for all the phenomena of anaesthesia. This may be the most desirable approach from the educational aspect, but the student simply has not got the time for it.

Some critics may carp at the somewhat colloquial style of the author. It is true that not all the periods are Johnsonian in character, but surely this is a good fault. It is all very well to describe the prognosis of delayed chloroform poisoning as 'the pathological changes and metabolic dysfunction are not infrequently so advanced as to become irreversible', but the student is much more likely to remember the gravity of the condition if he reads that 'it is usually fatal'.

Most textbooks are intolerably dull: this one is frequently amusing and for this reason alone should prove popular.

London 1949   C. Langton Hewer

Christopher Langton Hewer, MB, BS, FFARCS, MRCP, DA

Dr. Langton Hewer died on 28 January 1986 in his ninetieth year. He was Consulting Anaesthetist to St. Bartholomew's Hospital, London and had been Editor of *Anaesthesia*, the Journal of the Association of Anaesthetists of Great Britain and Ireland, for 20 years (1946–1966). Dr. Hewer was one of the great intellectual leaders of the specialty during the period of rapid development between the two World Wars and after World War II. He was a quiet and intimate man who preferred to exert his considerable influence from the background and with his pen but, as important, he was kind and considerate to the many trainees who passed through his hands and treated their indiscretions with tolerance salted with dry humour.

T.B.B.

Preface

'The most notable advance . . . . in my own surgical career has been in the field of anaesthesia'.

Manchester Medical Society 1954. Sir Heneage Ogilvie (1887–1971)

The first edition of this book was written in Auckland harbour during a dock strike in the New Zealand winter of 1948. Dr. Bryce-Smith stringently revised the texts of the third to the ninth editions, the original author being responsible for the editorial work. The present edition has been rewritten to meet the needs of clinical medical students in the 1980s, under the supervision of the two senior authors but with the aim of preserving its original character.

One of the junior members of the team gave his first solo anaesthetic for an obstetric emergency as a senior medical student in a London teaching hospital about the time the first edition was written. This was two or three weeks after completing the then obligatory one month of practical training in anaesthesia. The assumption of such a responsibility, natural at the time, would now be unacceptable. By contrast, 15 years later the most junior member of the team was initially heavily supervised for at least 3 months as a 'resident anaesthetist' (a houseman position now abolished with the upgrading of the specialty) before being allowed to give anaesthetics on his own. The medical student of 1948 was still trained as if he would be required to take the kind of clinical responsibility that might be demanded of a ship's doctor — including giving an anaesthetic and operating in an emergency — immediately after passing his final examination. The student of 1989 is given a broad view of medicine as a preliminary to specialisation after registration. Changes in the manner of presentation of *Anaesthetics for Medical Students* are therefore inevitable. The present volume is not a reference book or a handbook. It is designed to be read as an entity. A certain amount of dogmatism is inevitable in such a work, but an attempt has been made to express conventional opinion with some indication when there is room for doubt. Chapter 14 on cardiopulmonary resuscitation includes a section on basic life support in the first aid situation away from the hospital because of the practical importance of this subject.

Several explanatory figures have been introduced in this edition for the first time. They are the work of Peter Cull and Andrew Bezear of the Audiovisual Department of St. Bartholomew's Hospital, London and Lionel Williams of the Department of Medical Illustration, Royal Berkshire Hospital, Reading. Detailed illustrations of apparatus have been avoided; fascinating as they are, these are best learned under the practical tutelage of an instructor, or if this is not possible, from large texts or manufacturers' handbooks.

This edition, like its predecessors, is small enough to be carried in a brief case and may be studied between theatre cases, on a bus, or while awaiting the entrance of an unpunctual surgeon or lecturer. We hope that this edition reflects the theory and practice of the modern specialty of anaesthesia, and that nothing is painfully dated except some of the anecdotes.

Bromley, Oxford and Reading, 1989   Gordon Ostlere
Roger Bryce-Smith
Thomas Boulton
Colin Blogg

Contents

PART 1

Theory

1

Introductory

'I esteem it the office of a physician not only to restore health but to mitigate pain and dolours.'

Francis Bacon (1561–1626)

Modern western civilisations take for granted that pain should be controlled, and in particular that the pain of surgery should be abolished. This was not always so. Our ancestors regarded pain as inevitable and to be accepted as part of life. Philosophers and theologians throughout history have gone further and stressed the benefits of suffering pain with stoicism and fortitude to strengthen moral character. Down the ages many physicians and surgeons have attempted to relieve pain by herbal extracts and other means. Some, even in the nineteenth century following the introduction of surgical anaesthesia, still believed that the experience of pain during surgery was essential for subsequent healing.

Though the principles and substances necessary for the production of pharmacological anaesthesia had been known for some time, anaesthesia did not develop in the western world until humanitarian attitudes in the nineteenth century made the circumstances propitious.

The introduction of general anaesthesia

On 16 October 1846 at the Massachusetts General Hospital,

Boston, USA, the dentist William Green Morton (1819–1868) gave the first successful public demonstration of general anaesthesia for surgery using ether — a compound known to Paracelsus (1493–1541) (Appendix A).

It is not surprising that this first anaesthetic was given by a dentist or that dentistry should be closely associated with the introduction of anaesthesia. Dental extractions, for which Morton had used ether in private before the demonstration at the Massachusetts General Hospital, were among the few operations undertaken before the advent of pharmacological anaesthesia. Morton was not the first to employ inhalational general anaesthesia in man, nor was he the first to use ether for that purpose, but it was his demonstration which initiated the rapid and dramatic spread of the 'good news' throughout the world and sparked off a revolution in surgical practice.

Surgeons before Morton had been merely operating on body surface lesions or carrying out a limited number of more major operations amid scenes of indescribable carnage and agony; after Morton, and with the introduction of antiseptic and aseptic surgery, the previously inaccessible regions of the body — the abdomen, the brain, the thorax, and finally the heart itself — became accessible to the surgeon. Each step was necessarily accompanied by, and often dependent on, new developments in anaesthetic techniques.

The introduction of pharmacological local anaesthesia

Before Morton's demonstration of general anaesthesia, compression of nerve trunks and refrigeration were known to produce insensibility of parts of the limbs and trunk. Later, attempts were made to produce local anaesthesia for surgery by physical means as a safer alternative. Pharmacological local analgesia awaited appreciation of the surface analgesic effects of cocaine, a natural drug known to the natives of Peru for many centuries.

Von Anrep of Würtzburg suggested cocaine as a surface anaesthetic for urology and laryngology in 1880, but the event which spread worldwide knowledge of the discovery as rapidly as after Morton's first public exhibition of general anaesthesia was the demonstration at the Ophthalmological Congress in Heidelberg on 15th September 1884 by Dr Joseph Brettaner on behalf of Carl Koller (1858–1954) of Vienna, of the value of cocaine for operations on the eye. Injection of cocaine around nerves (using the syringe and hollow needle introduced by Alexander Wood of Edinburgh in 1885) originated in the USA in November of the same year.

Cocaine is a toxic and addictive drug, but synthetic alternatives, notably procaine, were shortly available, and alternative techniques as spinal anaesthesia (injection into the cerebro-spinal fluid) were soon developed (Appendix A).

The course of surgical history might have been very different had the discovery of pharmacological *local* anaesthesia preceded the discovery of pharmacological *general* anaesthesia. There is now a useful spectrum of anaesthetic techniques ranging from local to general anaesthesia via combinations of local and general anaesthetics.

The modern specialty of anaesthesia

The development of surgical anaesthesia sprang from a desire to abolish the pain of surgery, but the abolition of surgical pain is not the only, or even the primary responsibility of the modern physician anaesthetist. His duties in the operating theatre today are:

1. To keep the patient alive in the face of the assault of surgery;
2. To keep the patient free from pain;
3. To condition the patient for surgery.

Ideal operating conditions usually benefit the patient by promoting good surgery, but there are some occasions when the surgeon must be prepared to accept less than perfect conditions in the interests of the safety of the patient. Surgery can be practised on the cadaver, anaesthesia cannot.

This book is about physician anaesthetists and their management of surgical patients during operations, but modern anaesthetists have many responsibilities elsewhere. Their expertise in keeping patients alive during surgery has led to the extension of their activities into resuscitation and the intensive care of medical as well as surgical patients, and their special knowledge of pain control brings involvement in the relief of chronic pain. Anaesthetists are called upon to facilitate the work of most departments in the modern general hospital. Indeed anaesthesia is now the largest specialist clinical discipline in the British National Health Service.

The anaesthetist should always remember that he is sharing in the treatment of the patients of his medical and surgical colleagues and will take their opinions into account. He expects in turn that others will appreciate the problems and limitations of anaesthesia, and that they will present their patients to him in as good a condition as is practicable. A basic knowledge of anaesthesia is therefore important for all clinicians.

We hope that readers will find this volume both informative and helpful and that it will be an encouragement to some to devote their professional lives to the fascinating and comprehensive specialty of anaesthesia. No other medical discipline so constantly demands such moment-to-moment decisions in the management of unconscious or acutely ill patients. An anaesthetist must always be prepared to assess a situation rapidly and act quickly.[1]

[1] The need for the anaesthetist to keep his wits about him at all times is strikingly illustrated by the story of a London anaesthetist in the 1930's who, obviously deservedly, rose to the head of his profession. He was administering an anaesthetic to a young lady for a dental extraction one insupportably hot afternoon in August. The operation was in the surgery of a fashionable Harley Street dentist and the only onlooker was the young

lady's mother, who insisted on staying in the room. The anaesthetist had just established surgical anaesthesia when he was horrified to see the dentist drop at the foot of the chair, overcome by the heat. The mother thought the dentist was dead, screamed and fainted too. The anaesthetist was therefore presented within a few seconds with not one unconscious patient but with three. What should he do? Displaying appropriate confidence and coolness he promptly picked up a pair of dental forceps, removed the diseased tooth, turned off the anaesthetic, took a wet sponge and revived the dentist by pressing it on his neck, and brought round the mother by throwing the glass of antiseptic mouthwash over her face; then he left the trio to sort it out for themselves.

* The need for the anaesthetist to keep his wits about him at all times is strikingly illustrated by the story of a London anaesthetist in the 1930's who, obviously deservedly, rose to the head of his profession. He was administering an anaesthetic to a young lady for a dental extraction one insupportably hot afternoon in August. The operation was in the surgery of a fashionable Harley Street dentist and the only onlooker was the young

2

Jargon

'When I use a word', Humpty Dumpty said in a rather
scornful tone, 'it means just what I choose it to mean —
neither more nor less'.
Through the Looking Glass   Lewis Carroll (1832–1898)

Anaesthesia like other scientific disciplines has its technical
vocabulary. This has evolved haphazardly and, unfortunately,
is not always precise, and is sometimes confusing. The same
word can have several technical interpretations according to
its context, and may have an entirely different meaning from
its common use.

Anaesthesia

This term is derived from two Greek words which together
mean 'loss of feeling or feeling or sensation'. It is used in that
sense by neurologists to indicate a pathological absence of
feeling in part of the body. 'Anaesthesia' was also employed
by John Elliotson of the North London (now University
College) Hospital who used hypnosis to control the pain of
surgery early in the nineteenth century in the years immediately before the introduction of pharmacological general
anaesthesia.

The present technical use of the word 'anaesthesia'
(meaning 'pain relief for surgery'), is attributed to the literary

7

American physician Oliver Wendell Holmes (1809–1894), who applied it to Morton's discovery of 'etherisation' soon after its introduction. The word 'anaesthesia' if used alone today, usually means 'general' anaesthesia.

General anaesthesia implies that the patient has been rendered reversibly unconscious by drugs for the execution of a painful operative procedure.

'Inhalational', 'intravenous', 'intramuscular' and 'rectal' anaesthesia are subdivisions of general anaesthesia. The adjectives define the route by which the drugs are introduced into the body and thence via the blood stream to the brain.

Local anaesthesia (or 'local analgesia' — see below) implies anaesthesia of only portions of the body. The painfree patient will be conscious, unless a technique in which general anaesthesia is combined with local anaesthesia (Chapter 5) or sedation is used.

Regional anaesthesia, (or 'analgesia' — see below) is often used synonymously with 'local' anaesthesia. It is correctly employed only when a local anaesthetic is applied to nerves or to the spinal cord, remote from the area to be made insensitive. The techniques of local and regional anaesthesia are discussed in Chapter 12.

Analgesia

Analgesia means freedom from pain. It is used in three ways by present-day anaesthetists.

1. To define the process of rendering a *conscious* patient free from pain — an 'analgesic' drug has this property. Well known examples are aspirin or morphine, though, as we shall see, these two drugs act in different ways to produce pain relief.
2. 'Analgesia' is used by some authorities in preference to the word 'anaesthesia' to describe 'local' or 'regional' anaesthesia. This is an extension of the concept that the term

'analgesia' implies that a patient can be *conscious* but free from pain.

3. 'Analgesia' is also used by anaesthetists to imply suppression of the synapses in the central nervous system of the *unconscious* patient thus preventing somatic withdrawal reflexes and autonomic responses such as tachycardia. The use of the word 'analgesia' in this context is not strictly accurate, as you cannot relieve pain if the patient is already unconscious and not experiencing it, but it is less cumbersome than the alternative 'reflex suppression'. The description 'nociceptive' (capable of causing pain) can be applied both to a stimulus which results in pain in the conscious patient and one which causes reflex response in the unconscious patient, but the term 'painful stimulus' is often used loosely in this context whether the patient is conscious, and thus capable of experiencing pain, or not.

Hypnosis and narcosis

Hypnosis literally means 'the state of being asleep', but to the anaesthetist it has more technical meanings.

1. The state of deprivation of the critical faculties induced by hypnotism.

2. Pharmacological sleep from which the patient cannot be roused to consciousness by physical stimulus, but under which he may still react unconsciously by withdrawal or autonomic reflexes if he has not been given sufficient 'analgesia' as well.[1]

---

[1] Surgical anaesthesia implies that the patient is in a state of hypnosis but has also received enough analgesia to ensure that he will not react reflexly to the surgical stimulus. A patient often phonates or makes purposeful movements during the initial stages of anaesthesia (for example, as if trying to remove the face mask) though he is oblivious of his surroundings.

Hypnotic is a traditional description of any drug which will help the patient to sleep. Barbiturates have now been almost entirely replaced by various members of the benzodiazepine group, except in surgical anaesthesia.

Narcosis is a state of stupor produced by drugs, and is another term applied to pharmacological sleep. 'Narcosis' is more accurate than 'hypnosis'. The term 'narcotic' is also rather confusingly used for morphine-like drugs of addiction.

Muscular relaxation, which allows access to the body cavities can be obtained in many ways, for example, by central depression of the nervous system, by local anaesthesia of the peripheral nerves, or by blocking the neuromuscular junction. Any drug which causes muscle to relax could be called a 'muscle relaxant'; but this term is almost exclusively reserved for the group of drugs which block the chemical transmission of a nerve impulse at the neuromuscular junction. It is often abbreviated to 'relaxant'.

Sedatives, anxiolytics, tranquillisers and antidepressants

Sedation, may be used vaguely to imply anything from allaying anxiety to inducing near natural sleep with drugs. Although 'sedative' should strictly be applied only to the older agents such as phenobarbitone which allay anxiety by depressing the highest critical cerebral centres of the brain, it is also used loosely for the more modern anxiolytic agents.

Anxiolysis is a reduction in anxiety without necessarily producing sedation. *Tranquilliser,* describes a drug which acts at a lower level of the central nervous system than the cerebral cortex, in particular to those of the benzodiazepine group, like diazepam.

Many thousands of ambulant patients rely on regular oral doses of tranquillisers to help them face the stresses of life. Tranquillisers are used also for pre-anaesthetic medication for patients who are not in pain. Moderate doses of tranquillisers administered intravenously induce a state of 'conscious sedation', in which verbal contact is maintained but in which the anxious patient can easily be managed. Conscious sedation is used in dentistry to facilitate conservative treatment in anxious patients and to supplement local anaesthetic techniques for other forms of surgery.

Antidepressants and other anxiolytic agents, which alter the mood and mental reactions of patients, have revolutionised psychiatric management in recent years. Some, such as droperidol, have found uses in surgical anaesthesia, others, like amitriptyline, in chronic pain control. The monoamine oxidase inhibitors and the tricyclic agents cause undesirable effects when combined with certain drugs used in anaesthesia (Chapter 12).

A warning. All hypnotic sedatives, tranquillisers and antidepressants in large doses, will cause loss of consciousness, respiratory depression and abolition of protective reflexes with all the potential dangers that this implies. The difference between drugs commonly used for sedation and those used for the intravenous induction of anaesthesia is simply the therapeutic margin. It is, for example, relatively easy to keep a patient conscious and sedated with benzodiazepine such as diazepam but much more difficult with anaesthetic agents such as thiopentone and methohexitone.

Anaesthesia and anaesthetists

The science of anaesthesia is called 'anaesthesia', 'anaesthetics' or 'anaesthesiology'. The *ae* dipthong is omitted in the USA.

An '*anaesthetist*' is the individual who administers an anaesthetic. Anaesthetics have always been administered by medical or dental practitioners in the United Kingdom and most of the British Commonwealth; in these countries therefore the term 'anaesthetist' necessarily implies a medically or

dentally qualified anaesthetist. This is not so in other parts
of the world where besides physician and dentist anaesthetists
(USA, Anesthesiologists), 'nurse' and and 'technician' anaesthetists are employed and receive a variable amount of
training. Nurse and technician anaesthetists are nowadays
usually supervised by physician anaesthetists, particularly in
Scandinavia and the USA, but sometimes they are directed
by the surgeon.

'Nurse anaesthetists', who administer anaesthesia, are
distinct from 'anaesthetic nurses', who assist the anaesthetist
in a similar manner to the way in which an operating theatre
nurse assists the surgeon. Operating Department Assistants
(ODA) are technicians trained to assist anaesthetists.

3

Perception and prevention of pain

'We are more sensible of one little touch of the Surgeon's lancet than of twenty wounds with a sword in the heat of battle'.

Michel Eyquem de Montaigne (1533–1592)

Pain has obvious practical purposes. It warns against danger; it aids diagnosis; it can sometimes promote healing by limiting movement and enforcing the immobilisation of an injured part. But, in surgery, once the diagnosis has been made, pain has no further purpose and should be eliminated.

The perception of pain

Pain is appreciated by the conscious patient at the highest critical levels of the cortex, but a peripheral stimulus is not necessarily interpreted as painful even in the absence of drugs.[1] It is well known that sportsmen on the playing field

[1] The importance of mental attitude was noted by Professor H. K. Beecher (the first Professor of Anesthesia at the Massachusetts General Hospital, Boston, USA) while he was serving in the US Army in World War II. Beecher observed that soldiers wounded in battle, who were in hospital and honourably out of the firing line with the knowledge of duty well done and the prospect of returning home, required less morphine for pain relief than the victims of automobile accidents in civilian life with all the worry of loss of earnings, possible prosecution and litigation looming before them.

13

and soldiers in battle can sustain remarkably severe injuries without realising that they have done so, because they are distracted by the excitement of the moment. It is also often possible to insert a needle painlessly into the vein of a child while the nurse distracts his attention.

The somatic reflex withdrawal reaction to pain can also be obtunded by inhibition from the higher centres. (Compare your own reaction to stepping unexpectedly on a drawing pin with a bare foot to your stoical acceptance of the similar stimulus of a therapeutic intramuscular injection . . .).

These and other phenomena associated with the appreciation of pain and its suppression can be related to the anatomy of the central nervous system. The electrical signal which transmits pain originates at the periphery, where tissue damage releases chemical substances which stimulate the nerve endings and the effect is potentiated by prostaglandins. The impulse passes through a multitude of synaptic relays on its way from the periphery to the cortex, initiating somatic and visceral reflex phenomena as it does so. If we aim to control the pain, we can block or modify the passage of the painful impulse through these relays by physical, psychological or physiological means, or by drugs, and inhibit the systemic and autonomic reflex phenomena at the same time.

Pain pathways

The spinal 'gate'. The impulse from a painful stimulus at the periphery is conducted by the nonmyelinated C fibres or the myelinated A fibres and relays first in the spinal cord in the substantia gelatinosa of the dorsal horn (Fig. 3.1). If the stimulus is sudden and unexpected it will pass through the relay or 'gate' mediated by the peptide neurotransmitter 'Substance P', and pass upwards in the cord towards the brain along the spinothalamic tracts. It may also initiate a withdrawal-type spinal reflex involving muscular contraction. The spasm thus engendered adds to the pain.

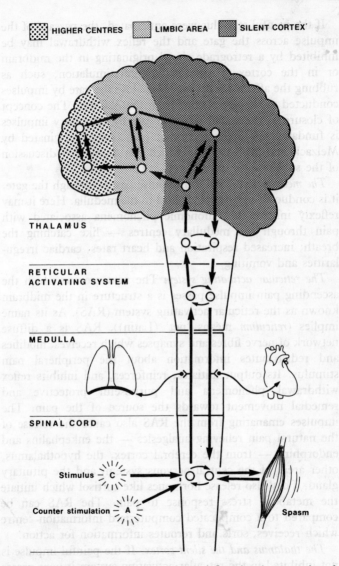

HIGHER CENTRES   LIMBIC AREA   'SILENT CORTEX'

THALAMUS

RETICULAR
ACTIVATING SYSTEM

MEDULLA

SPINAL CORD

Stimulus — C

Counter stimulation — A

Spasm

Fig. 3.1 Afferent and efferent pain pathways influencing the perception of pain (see text).

If the painful stimulus were anticipated, the passage of the impulse across the gate and the reflex withdrawal may be inhibited by a retrograde signal originating in the midbrain or in the cortex. Peripheral counterstimulation, such as rubbing the affected area, may also close the gate by impulses conducted to the spinal cord from the A fibres. The concept of closure of the spinal synaptic gate by inhibitory impulses is fundamental to the theory of pain control originated by Melzack and Wall in 1965 which has dominated discussion of the subject ever since.

The medulla If the painful impulse passes through the gate, it is conducted up the spinal cord to the medulla. Here it may reflexly initiate the autonomic phenomena associated with pain through the medullary centres — like catching the breath; increased respiration and heart rates; cardiac irregularities and vomiting.

The reticular activating system The next area to which the ascending pain impulse passes is a structure in the midbrain known as the reticular activating system (RAS). As its name implies (*reticulum* means 'net' (Latin)), RAS is a diffuse network of nerve fibres and synapses which receives, modifies and redistributes information about the peripheral pain stimulus. Its output initiates, reinforces, and inhibits reflex withdrawal phenomena and purposeful protective and remedial movement towards the source of the pain. The impulses emanating from the RAS also cause the release of the natural pain relieving analgesics — the enkephalins and endorphins — from the cerebral cortex, the hypothalamus, other areas of the central nervous system, and the pituitary gland. They also release hormones like cortisol which initiate the metabolic stress response to pain. The RAS can be compared to a complicated computerised information centre which receives, sorts and reroutes information for action.

The thalamus and the silent cortex. If the painful impulse is not inhibited in the reticular activating system it next passes to the thalamus. Pain is coarsely appreciated in this developmentally ancient part of the brain. It then also passes to the 'silent' somatosensory cortex, where it is assessed, localised and stored in the memory.

The limbic system is the connecting structure which leads to the frontal cortex — here the immediate emotional response to pain is generated.

The frontal cortex finally appreciates the impulse as pain and consciously initiates discriminatory emotional and physical reactions to combat its cause.

The psychological and physical control of pain in the conscious patient

Much can be done to inhibit pain by psychological and physical mechanisms without resort to drugs.

Suggestion and distraction. We have already noted how sympathy and suggestion at the highest cortical level, and their extension in the form of hypnosis can distract the patient from appreciating pain. The pain impulse is prevented from getting through to the cortex; rather like dialling a telephone number which is already engaged.

Massive sensory input — for example, auditory stimuli in the form of music or 'white' sound (sound of multiple frequencies) applied by earphones can so 'occupy' the synapses of the limbic system, thalamus and reticular activating system that the appreciation of pain is inhibited.

Acupuncture — simple mechanical manipulation and low frequency electric stimulation of the needles distracts the patient as well as releasing endogenous enkephalins and endorphins to block the opiate receptors.

Counterstimulation. We have already discussed the closure of the spinal gate by impulses transmitted from the periphery by sensory myelinated A nerve fibres, from simple mechanical actions like rubbing the affected part. In the nineteen thirties

children were brought up in a world in which medical counterstimulation by comforting liniments, camphorated oil,
poultices, ice packs, etc., played an important part in
therapy. A modern extension of such treatment is the aerosol
cold spray for sportsmen's sprains, and transcutaneous nerve
stimulation (TNS), used to alleviate chronic pain, by means
of a continuously applied low frequency electric shock.

The control of pain by drugs

There are a number of pharmacological substances which can
be used as 'analgesics' to relieve pain in the conscious patient
without producing the total oblivion of general anaesthesia.

Simple sedatives, such as the oral barbiturates, can dull the
perception of pain at the cortical level in the conscious
patient. This is really stage 1 anaesthesia and is considered
in more detail in Chapter 5.

Tranquillisers such as the benzodiazepine diazepam, act on
the limbic area and control the emotional response to pain.

Opioid analgesics are the most useful pain relievers. They
act on receptors which are widely distributed throughout the
brain and spinal cord. Some, like pethidine, exert their effect
almost exclusively in the midbrain and spinal cord on those
synapses which control analgesia. Others, including morphine,
also act at higher levels on receptors which modify attitudes
to pain, and may produce euphoria. They may have
unwanted side effects in the medulla by stimulating the
vomiting centre and depressing the respiratory centre.

Phenothiazines depress the reticular activating system. They
generally enhance the effect of analgesics and other drugs
acting on the area. They reduce the onward transmission of
signals from the periphery which keeps the cortex in a state
of aroused activity; thus they have a tranquillising and
anxiolytic effect, and so potentiate tranquillisers, sedatives
and anaesthetics acting on the higher centres. The phenothi-

azines centrally inhibit the sympathetic nervous system, causing vasodilation. They are antiemetics through selective action on the medullary vomiting centre.

Local anaesthetics can be applied to the spinal cord, to nerve roots, and to the peripheral nerves to prevent painful impulses from reaching the spinal cord — examples are epidural blocks in routine obstetric delivery and intercostal nerve blocks to obtund the pain of fractured ribs.

Antiprostaglandin analgesics (aspirin, paracetamol, etc.) act at the source of the pain by preventing the formation of prostaglandins which increase the excitability of pain nerve endings. They are particularly useful when respiratory depression must be avoided, and if there is likely to be much inflammation.

Inhalational agents Some inhaled anaesthetic agents may produce analgesia when used in concentrations too low for unconsciousness to result. Trichlorethylene and methoxyflurane delivered in limited concentration from accurately calibrated vaporizers, have been used extensively in obstetric and traumatic pain relief. Nitrous oxide 50% in oxygen has become widely available premixed in cylinders as 'Entonox' (Ohmeda Ltd.) or supplied by a central piped source. Patients are asked to hold the mask to their faces themselves so that it falls away before sufficient gas is inhaled to produce unconsciousness.

Pain control and the surgical patient

All these psychological, physical and pharmacological processes which modify, reduce or eliminate the appreciation of pain, have their uses in the alleviation of the pain of the surgical patient, whether preoperatively, during surgery itself as part of the anaesthetic technique, or in the postoperative period.

4

The action of drugs

'Action is transitory . . . the motion of a muscle this way or
that'.
The Borderers   William Wordsworth (1770–1850)

Pharmacodynamics: the actions of the drugs used in surgical anaesthesia

Pharmacodynamics is the study of the effect of drugs on the
body. The result of administering the drugs used by anaesthetists is usually almost immediately obvious but the detailed
mechanisms by which they act may not yet be fully elucidated.

Pharmacokinetics considers what the body does to drugs.
Their uptake, distribution, biotransformation and elimination, and the particular cells on which they act determines
rapidity of onset, length of action, toxicity, side effects, etc.

How do the drugs used in general anaesthesia act? Many
groups of drugs are used in modern surgical anaesthesia. The
action of each group is broadly discussed below; later, principally in Chapter 8, we shall consider individual drugs and
how they can be combined to the best advantage.

Drugs acting on the central nervous system (general anaesthetics, sedatives, tranquilisers and analgesics) can be introduced into the body by several routes (intravenous,
intramuscular, inhalational, oral, rectal, sublingual, and
transdermal[1].

Whatever the route of introduction, all anaesthetics pass into the bloodstream and are transported to the brain, where they penetrate the blood–brain barrier and enter specific cells in the central nervous system (CNS). Here they exert their characteristic reversible effects but the precise mechanisms are not fully understood. It is probable that the anaesthetic state is caused by an alteration in the permeability of the brain cell membrane, and possibly interference with oxygenation, intracellular hydrogen ion concentration and/or ion exchange. Various mechanisms have been suggested, including reversible distortion of the protein elements of the membrane and blocking of the sodium channels. The interesting experimental finding that increasing the hydrostatic pressure around a small organism (e.g. a tadpole) can reverse the action of pharmacological anaesthetics — possibly by correcting the altered membrane permeability by a pressure effect, and 'squeezing' it back into its normal shape, supports the theory of membrane distortion.

Centrally acting drugs act on specific receptors in the brain. Opioid analgesics have several different types of receptors scattered throughout the brain and spinal cord. Each is specific for the various clinical effects that characterise individual opioids.

General anti-inflammatory analgesics. These agents include aspirin and paracetamol. They are usually administered by mouth, but after absorption into the bloodstream, act locally at the periphery of the traumatic swelling or inflammation by inhibiting the synthesis of pain enhancing prostaglandins.

Local anaesthetics are injected or applied topically close to the cell or to the axonal nerve process on which they are to

---

[1] Veterinary surgeons and research workers use intraperitoneal injection to produce anaesthesia in animals with barbiturates and other drugs; this is not used in humans. In the "play within a play" in *Hamlet* an overdose of a soporific drug is adminstered via the external meatus of the ear. This method finds little favour in present medical practice!

act. They penetrate the axonal or cell membrane, exert their blocking action, and are later absorbed into the bloodstream, destroyed and eliminated.

The mechanism of action of locally applied anaesthetic agents is better understood than general anaesthesia. Local anaesthetics are composed of aromatic and tertiary amine groups linked by a group which is either an ester or an amide. One end of the molecule is lipophilic which, in the relatively alkaline milieu around the nerve, enables the local anaesthetic to penetrate the lipoid membrane of the nerve axon. The inside of the nerve is relatively acid and this leads to the release of the ionised form of the local anaesthetic. This then blocks the sodium channels in the nerve cell membrane, and thus prevents the ionic exchange essential for the normal transmission of the electrical impulse along the axon.

The greater the protein binding capacity of a local anaesthetic agent the longer its action.

Neuromuscular blocking agents ('muscle relaxants'). Transmission of the nerve impulse to the muscle at the neuromuscular junction of voluntary muscle is accomplished by acetylcholine. Small amounts of acetylcholine are repeatedly released at rest. Larger amounts are released when an impulse is conducted down the motor nerve fibre to the nerve ending. The acetylcholine crosses, the myoneural junctional cleft and becomes attached to the paired lipoprotein receptors grouped around ion channels in the membrane. This makes the membrane of the muscle endplate permeable to an inward flow of sodium and calcium ions and the exit of intracellular potassium ions. Depolarisation thus occurs, an electrical potential is produced and propagated, and the muscle contracts. The acetylcholine is then rapidly hydrolysed by acetylcholinesterase, which is present in the vicinity of the motor-end plate. The products are then taken up again by the nerve ending and resynthesized into acetylcholine, and the neuromuscular junction repolarises and awaits the next impulse.

There are two types of muscle relaxants.

Depolarisers, typified by suxamethonium, act similarly to acetylcholine by causing depolarisation, but instead of repolarisation occurring immediately, the depolarisation persists and the muscle remains flaccid until the relaxant is destroyed by another enzyme (serum-or 'pseudo'-cholinesterase). The action of a depolarising muscle relaxant is 'all-or-nothing', because a single molecule of depolarising drug attaching itself to a single endplate receptor will trigger the total response of depolarisation for that muscle fibre. Depolarising neuromuscular agents are not reversible by neostigmine under normal circumstances (see below). Indeed, neostigmine may prolong the depolarising block by flooding the endplate with acetylcholine which is not destroyed because the acetylcholinesterase enzyme is inhibited.

Nondepolarisers or competitive blocking agents. These are typified by tubocurarine chloride. Nondepolarisers occupy the endplate receptors without causing depolarisation, and thus deny all or some of the receptors to the natural transmitter acetylcholine. The overall effect of nondepolarisers will, therefore, depend on how many receptors are occupied. Weakened rather than paralysed muscle will result if some acetylcholine molecules still manage to occupy some receptors. Nondepolarising block is reversed by neostigmine. This drug inhibits the acetylcholinesterase, so the local concentration of acetylcholine increases which then competes for the receptors and reverses the neuromuscular block. The nondepolarising agent is then removed in the bloodstream and excreted or destroyed. Normal neuromuscular transmission is thus restored.

5

Classical and modern concepts

> 'There is occasions and causes why and wherefore in all things.'
> Fluellen in *King Henry V*. Act V scene i.
> William Shakespeare (1564–1616)

Pharmacological local anaesthesia was not introduced until 1884 — nearly forty years after Morton's first successful public demonstration of the use of ether. There is sometimes a tendency to regard local and general anaesthesia as alternatives, but there is a spectrum of techniques available to anaesthetists.

1. Local anaesthesia alone;
2. Local anaesthesia with pharmacological sedation.
3. Local anaesthesia combined with general anaesthesia.
4. General anaesthesia alone, with and without paralysis by neuromuscular blocking agents and controlled ventilation.

British anaesthetists predominantly favour general anaesthesia, but careful assessment of the indications for general, local or combined techniques should be made in each case.

A radical change occurred with the introduction of the muscle relaxants in 1942 by Griffith and Johnson and the development of their use with elective controlled ventilation of the paralysed patient by Gray and Halton (1946) (Appendix A). An alternative technique was thus created for producing abdominal muscular relaxation without the potential hazards of spontaneous respiration during deep general anaesthesia.

The classic general anaesthetic

The aim of modern polypharmaceutical general anaesthesia is to produce unconsciousness quickly with an intravenous agent and then to maintain a depth of anaesthesia appropriate for the surgery. The reasons for this and the techniques employed are discussed later. Anaesthesia with an inhalational agent is nowadays only rarely pressed to the stage of medullary depression, and it might therefore seem irrelevant to discuss the stages of deep ether anaesthesia and the signs that accompany them. We make no apology for doing so, because much that follows can best be understood if related to classic ether anaesthesia.

It was fortunate for early success and acceptance of anaesthesia that ether is a safe and effective inhalational anaesthetic. This is because:

1. It is a sympathomimetic agent which preserves cardiac output and blood pressure and yet causes few cardiac irregularities.
2. Induction and increasing the depth of anaesthesia with ether alone is a gradual process easily monitored. Ether being readily soluble in blood it is only slowly released to the brain.
3. Adequate abdominal relaxation for surgery can be obtained by ether alone with the patient breathing spontaneously. Depression of the medullary respiratory centre to the point of apnoea only occurs with extremely deep ether anaesthesia. This is in contrast to the effect of more modern inhalational agents like halothane, enflurane, and isoflurane or to intravenous drugs including thiopentone.

Induction is certainly gradual with ether, but recovery from deep ether anaesthesia is lingering because of the slow elimination of the large volumes dissolved in the blood. The effects of unnecessarily prolonged postoperative immobilis-ation, such as hypostatic pneumonia and deep vein throm-bosis, cause morbidity and sometimes death. Although the pioneer anaesthetists saw no alternative to deep anaesthesia to produce adequate relaxation for abdominal surgery, they also sought to use only light anaesthesia for superficial oper-ations such as the extraction of teeth or the incision of abscesses, to avoid the consequences of prolonged recovery. It was therefore essential for them to assess the depth of anaesthesia as accurately as possible, and consequently, detailed studies were made of the signs accompanying the gradually deepening stages of anaesthesia.

The stages of anaesthesia

The stages or levels of anaesthesia have been defined as 'awake, asleep, dead' by a cynical senior anaesthetist. An earlier discerning practitioner, John Snow[1], described the transition from consciousness to deep etherisation as the 'five stages of narcotism', but the most generally accepted classi-fication is that of Arthur Guedel (1883–1956), Professor of Anesthesiology at the University of Southern California[2].

[1] John Snow (1813–1858) who was born in York and worked in London, was the first medical man to practice anaesthesia as a specialty. He had a fertile and logical mind and achieved the first truly scientific approach to the subject. He practised the administration of ether soon after its introduction to England at the end of 1846. He is remembered for his scholarly books and for his administration of chloroform to Queen Victoria at the birth of Prince Leopold, in 1853. This event ended the theological controversy as to whether or not the admonition of Jehovah to woman at the time of the expulsion from the Garden of Eden — 'in sorrow shalt thou bring forth children' — was a divine command which excluded the use of pain relief in childbirth.

[2] Guedel's four stages of general anaesthesia are very naturally not dissimilar to those of alcohol intoxication — 1. Dizzy and Delightful: 2. Disorientated and Destructive: 3. Dead Drunk: 4. Danger of Dying. Fortunately few social drinkers get further than Stage 1 anaesthesia.

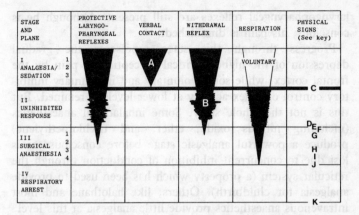

STAGE AND PLANE	PROTECTIVE LARYNGO-PHARYNGEAL REFLEXES	VERBAL CONTACT	WITHDRAWAL REFLEX	RESPIRATION	PHYSICAL SIGNS (See key)
I ANALGESIA/ SEDATION 1 2 3		A		VOLUNTARY	C
II UNINHIBITED RESPONSE			B		D E F G
III SURGICAL ANAESTHESIA 1 2 3 4					H I J
IV RESPIRATORY ARREST					K

Fig. 5.1 Guedel's classical signs of ether anaesthesia (see text).
A = Verbal communication and voluntary response throughout Stage I.
B = Reflex and purposeful but unconscious movements throughout Stage II. C = Loss of consciousness. D = Active vomiting reflex obtunded.
E = Regular automatic breathing. Eyelid reflex goes. F = Swallowing ceases. Visceral reflexes obtunded. G = Eye movement ceases. Reaction to skin incision disappears. H = Respiration becomes jerky and diaphragmatic 'Tracheal Tug' develops. I = Carinal reflex disappears J = Respiration ceases K = Cardiac arrest.

General anaesthesia has been described as the depression of the central nervous system from the highest centres downwards. This is only broadly true. Reference to Figure 3.1 will help in understanding the concept of these stages. Figure 5.1 illustrates the accompanying signs of increasing depth of anaesthesia which were described primarily for patients who were spontaneously inhaling ether without narcotic supplements.

Stage 1 — the stage of analgesia extends from the start of the inhalational induction to loss of consciousness. The patient remains in verbal contact and accessible to reassurance and suggestion throughout this stage of anaesthesia. He can make voluntary purposeful movements and the protective laryngopharyngeal reflexes are still present. Although he is conscious, his pain is diminished.

Progress through this stage represents the gradual depression of the highest critical perception of pain by the frontal cortex, while some voluntary and involuntary inhibitory control of reflex activity at lower levels is retained. But this is not the whole story. Some inhalational anaesthetics (including nitrous oxide, ether, and trichloroethylene) produce a powerful analgesic stage before consciousness is lost due to concurrent inhibition of conduction through the reticular system (a property which has been used to provide analgesia for childbirth). Others, like halothane and most intravenous anaesthetics provide little analgesia at this level.

Stage 1 has gained increased importance in recent years as the stage used, with or without local anaesthesia, by dental surgeons in the technique known as 'relative analgesia', which uses nitrous oxide for pain control during conservative dental procedures. The maintenance of verbal contact is an important sign, present so long as the patient is conscious and the vital laryngopharyngeal reflexes are not unduly diminished (Figure 5.1 and see below). The British General Dental Council ruled in 1983 that the use of Stage 1 analgesia by operating dental surgeons working with trained paramedical assistants was acceptable. Some of those who use relative analgesia divide Stage 1 (the stage of analgesia) into three or more planes as the effect of the anaesthetic agent increases.

Stage 2. The stage of uninhibited response is often incorrectly called the 'stage of excitement'. This is an understandable misnomer. The stage begins when the highest cortical centres are fully depressed. The patient therefore loses consciousness, verbal contact goes, and with it voluntary control. The last remnants of higher cortical control of the mid brain by the cortex are thus removed, and the patient becomes a prey to uncontrolled, exaggerated, withdrawal type response to almost any stimulus (Figure 5.1). Consequently breathing may be irregular, there may be breath holding, apparently purposeful and uncoordinated limb movement, phonation, coughing, and laryngeal spasm from even small amounts of saliva stimulating the protective reflexes of the larynx. At this stage active vomiting may, and often did, occur in prolonged inhalational ether inductions — it was therefore fortunate that the protective laryngopharyngeal reflexes remained at this level of anaesthesia.

The stage of uninhibited response was notorious in the past in both fact and fable.[3] Nowadays only the remnants of this phase remain. The patient can be anaesthetised rapidly with intravenous drugs and the newer inhalational agents like halothane and enflurane, and quiet conditions exist for super-vised recovery.

Stage 3. Surgical anaesthesia is the stage during which operations may be performed while the patient is both obli-vious and incapable of interfering by reflex action. It is the stage at which anaesthesia has depressed both the reticular activating system and, perhaps selectively, the pain synapses of the spinal cord (Fig. 3.1). The centres of the medulla become progressively depressed. These include the vomiting centre (so that active vomiting is no longer a danger), the centres maintaining striated muscle tone — including that of the abdominal wall — and the respiratory centre. Autonomic responses, such as reflex quickening or slowing of the heart, or respiration from visceral stimuli (pulling on the mesentery of the guts etc.), are depressed comparatively early in surgical

[3] This was particularly so in dental outpatient departments and surgeries where, in the short time available with nitrous oxide as it was administered by junior and occasional anaesthetists, the dental surgeon might stimulate the patient by attempting to extract teeth in the induction or recovery phases. The burly manual worker fighting in the 'excitation' phase was someone to be reckoned with. The presence of a muscular *custos mas* (male attendant) in Hospital outpatient departments was an essential part of the dental outpatient team until the introduction of intravenous induction and halothane in the late 1950's.

anaesthesia, but with ether, spontaneous respiration does not cease until the anaesthesia is deep. Indeed, Guedel defined surgical anaesthesia as between the point at which respiration was no longer influenced by reflex stimuli and became regular, and the point at which respiration ceased because of medullary depression.

Deep etherisation was necessary for adequate abdominal muscular relaxation. The administrators of traditional spontaneously respired ether anaesthetics for upper abdominal surgery were compelled to steer a narrow course between achieving satisfactory relaxation of the abdominal wall and stopping the patient breathing. Stage 3 surgical anaesthesia was therefore divided into four planes defining the state of etherisation at which body surface, lower abdominal, and upper abdominal operations could be undertaken. Anaesthetists were trained to relate the depth of anaesthesia to a number of reflex physical signs, some of these and the levels they matched are indicated in Figure 5.1.

Stage 4. The stage of respiratory arrest (or, more crudely, of 'danger of death') extended from the cessation of spontaneous respiration to the point at which anoxia and the direct effect of the anaesthetic caused cardiac arrest. The gap between these two events was fortunately considerable with ether, but it was narrow or non-existent with chloroform. Ventricular fibrillation could also occur under light chloroform anaesthesia because it sensitised the heart to the circulating adrenaline of the frightened patient. Today, when respiratory paralysis is commonly produced with neuromuscular blocking relaxants and ventilation is electively controlled (see below), it is difficult for us to appreciate how gravely former generations of anaesthetists regarded respiratory arrest.

Modern techniques of general anaesthesia

Modern techniques of general anaesthesia aim to keep the

patient in light surgical anaesthesia equivalent to plane 2 of ether Stage 3 anaesthesia, from which recovery is rapid. Abdominal muscle relaxation is provided by peripherally acting drugs (local anaesthetics or neuromuscular blocking agents) when it is required. These drugs also inhibit nociceptive and stretch reflexes arising at the periphery. There are thus fewer 'arousal' reflexes arriving at the cortex and only minimal amount of general anaesthetic is given to ensure unconsciousness.[4]

Balanced anaesthesia. The idea of avoiding unnecessarily deep anaesthesia by using drugs other than general anaesthetics to produce muscular relaxation and reflex suppression originated in the teachings of the American surgeon George Washington Crile (1864–1943) at the beginning of the century. He used local anaesthesia in combination with general anaesthesia. The concept of balanced anaesthesia was developed and extended by Professor T. Cecil Gray of Liverpool using muscle relaxants. Gray described anaesthesia as being composed of three components — 'narcosis' (pharmacological sleep), 'reflex suppression' (or analgesia) and muscular 'relaxation' each of which could, and should be, controlled separately.

Light general anaesthesia alone with the patient breathing spontaneously is used for body surface surgery, minor orthopaedic procedures, minor vaginal gynaecological surgery and endoscopic investigations like cystoscopy and sigmoidoscopy, for which profound muscular paralysis is unnecessary.

The patient should be in the equivalent of Stage 3 ether anaesthesia somewhere between Plane 1 and Plane 2. He is usually taken rapidly through Stages 1 and 2 by an intravenous

---

[4] The cerebral cortex is regarded by some as being asleep unless it is 'aroused' by peripheral stimuli of one kind or another, but the student should be warned that this simplistic interpretation appeals to the anaesthetist rather than the neurophysiologist.

induction agent like thiopentone. The anaesthetic is generally maintained by spontaneously inhaling an agent such
as halothane, enflurane or isoflurane. It is unlikely that the
anaesthesia will become too deep because respiratory
depression occurs at a light plane of anaesthesia with these
modern agents and the anaesthetist can hardly ignore this
sign. Recovery will be rapid when the inhalation anaesthetic
is withdrawn, as the agents in use today are relatively insol-
uble in blood, and are therefore quickly eliminated. The risk
of the patient becoming aware during a spontaneously
respired inhalation anaesthetic is virtually unknown with this
technique.

*Light spontaneously respired general anaesthesia with local
anaesthesia.* Local anaesthesia combined with general anaesthesia has been regaining popularity during the last few years,
but it is surprising that the technique was not generally
popular with anaesthetists and surgeons before the introduction of muscle relaxants, as it offers a method of avoiding
deep general anaesthesia for abdominal surgery while
providing oblivion for the patient and allowing relatively
rapid recovery[5].

Some authorities today believe that *all* major spinal
subarachnoid and epidural procedures for abdominal surgery
should be 'covered' by light general anaesthesia for humanitarian reasons. These techniques block the autonomic visceral

---

[5] One reason for the apparent disregard of this important method may
be that its originator, Crile, was not primarily concerned with promoting a
technique from which recovery from anaesthesia was rapid. Crile was
interested in preventing 'shock'. He believed that 'shock' was caused by
the bombardment of the brain by neurogenic 'nociceptive' stimuli from the
site of the operation, and he sought to abolish such stimuli by regional
blockade with procaine. Though it is now recognised that surgical 'shock'
is most usually due to hypovolaemia, it is interesting that regional
analgesia covering the operative area has been shown to block the release
of cortisol and other hormones in response to surgery, and reduce their
undesirable cardiac and metabolic effects.

efferent nerves, as well as eliminating pain and providing excellent muscular relaxation by somatic motor nerve block.

The introduction of the longer acting reversible local anaesthetics as bupivacaine has further extended the value of combined local and general anaesthesia as pain relief continues into the early postoperative period after the patient has regained consciousness.

Light general anaesthesia with neuromuscular block. The revolution caused in the 1940's by the introduction of neuromuscular blocking agents was dramatic, but the real advance was the development of the combination of complete paralysis of the muscles of respiration, with the deliberate use of endotracheal intubation and controlled ventilation.[6] It must be confessed that the early practice of attempting to secure adequate abdominal relaxation by using neuromuscular blocking agents while maintaining satisfactory spontaneous respiration, though successfully achieved by some, led to many deaths from asphyxia.[7]

The amount of general anaesthetic agent required to keep the patient unconscious is less when ventilation is controlled than when breathing is spontaneous. Why should this be? If we accept the arousal theory, it can be argued that once the incision is made in an abdominal operation, and the knife is deeper than the network of sensitive nerve endings immediately beneath the skin, the main arousal stimuli will be stretch impulses as the retractors pull the muscles apart (Figure 3.1).

---

[6] The elements which make up the modern muscle relaxant-intubation-controlled ventilation technique were known for an astonishingly lengthy period by physiologists and others before its use in man. (Appendix A).

[7] This was particularly the case in North America where the 'extraordinary' British practice of administering large doses of muscle relaxants, intubating and controlling ventilation, and then reversing the relaxant with neostigmine, was finally only accepted after considerable mortality from the use of curare with spontaneous respiration.

If muscle tone is completely abolished there will be no bombardment of the brain with stretch impulses, and the amount of anaesthetic required to keep the patient unconscious by depression of the cerebrum will be reduced. Moderate hyperventilation reduces the blood carbon dioxide tension (to 4 kPa or less from the normal 5.3 kPa) and this also makes the brain more sensitive to general anaesthetics. The fall in cerebral blood flow resulting from hypocarbia in elderly patients may be responsible for occasional postoperative confusion.

Care must be taken to administer enough anaesthesia or the patient may become 'aware', and suffer the terrifying experience of knowing he is being operated upon but is paralysed and unable to attract the attention of the anaesthetist. So long as awareness is avoided, however, the controlled ventilation and muscle relaxant technique has the advantage of light anaesthesia, assured oxygen and carbon dioxide elimination, profound abdominal muscular relaxation and rapid recovery of consciousness.

The controlled ventilation technique has also solved the problem of the surgically induced pneumothorax in thoracic anaesthesia, and has advantages in other specialties, including ophthalmic and paediatric practice. It is the only truly universal technique of anaesthesia which can be used for every type of operation, (including body surface, abdominal and thoracic procedures) in almost any environment.

The disadvantages (in addition to the dangers of failure to intubate and awareness) are, absolute dependence on properly supervised and administered controlled ventilation, the possibility of prolonged total or partial paralysis from muscle relaxants, and less drastically, sore throat and effects on the trachea of intubation, a necessary part of the technique.

Total intravenous anaesthesia (TIVA) is a technique designed to induce and maintain general anaesthesia by intravenous agents alone. Interest in total intravenous anaesthesia has been stimulated since the importance of avoiding atmospheric pollution with inhalation agents has been recognised. Induction is usually by bolus injection of a drug, and then maintenance by continuous infusion. Patients maintained by TIVA breathing spontaneously tend to move suddenly if anaesthesia is too light, and to stop breathing if it is too deep. TIVA is most appropriate when used with muscle relaxants and controlled ventilation. Althesin and etomidate infusions were proven to be useful TIVA agents but their withdrawal because of side effects has resulted in a decline in the use of TIVA techniques. Newer agents, such as propofol, offer hope of a return to popularity of the total intravenous technique.

The use of local anaesthesia for conscious patients

Minor surgery. Much minor surgery can be undertaken under local anaesthesia. It is probably used less often than it should in United Kingdom practice, especially in outpatient departments. Local analgesia has advantages of rapid recovery and low systemic morbidity, but it has a definite failure rate. Patients and medical and nursing staff alike often prefer the certainty of general anaesthesia, and the incidence of the minor morbid effects of recovery have become acceptable and less important with the newer intravenous and inhalational agents. The British National Health Service also tries to ensure that skilled physician anaesthetists are readily available and thus the risks of general anaesthesia are minimised.

The success of techniques of local analgesia can be greatly increased by constant use, so that medical, nursing and paramedical personnel are familiar with the procedures, by careful psychological management of the patients, and by supplementary sedative and analgesic medication including low concentrations of nitrous oxide.

Major surgery. General anaesthesia always imposes an additional risk, however small, even in skilled hands, but major surgery is usually better undertaken without having continuously to reassure the anxious conscious patient. General anaesthesia is often considered to be mandatory in cardiothoracic, neurological and neonatal surgery.

Sometimes local anaesthesia has distinct advantages, for example in obstetric anaesthesia and for elderly patients for urological and orthopaedic operations. Patients in their eighties and nineties are reputed to suffer some deterioration of mental faculties after surgery and general anaesthesia. This may only be detectable to their relatives ('Grandma was never quite the same after her anaesthetic'). The adverse effects of anaesthesia are often impossible to separate from those from changes in environment, the surgical pathology, the use of analgesics, and the metabolic or physiological upset involved.

PART 2

Practice

6

Safety first

'It's dangerous to take cold, to sleep, to drink, but I tell you my Lord fool, out of this nettle, danger, we pluck this flower, safety'
Hotspur in *Henry IV, Part 1*. Act II sc.iii.
William Shakespeare (1584–1616)

We emphasised in Chapter 1 that the first duty of the anaesthetist is to keep the patient alive during surgery. He should always remember that anaesthesia is not an end in itself. The ideal anaesthetic would present no risk to the life or the wellbeing of the patient (or for that matter to operating theatre personnel), but this is an impossibility. Both general and local anaesthetics are dangerous drugs. The state of unconsciousness is itself hazardous, and apparatus can fail unexpectedly. The best that can be done is to ensure that the risk to the patient is minimal. Danger is reduced if the relevant history is obtained and the patient is carefully examined and prepared for anaesthesia, but the unexpected cannot always be avoided (for example the response of individual subjects to specific drugs is very variable) and vigilance is vital both during and after anaesthesia.

The preparation of the patient[1]

1. *Routine preparation* is undertaken to ensure that the

patient is in the best physical and physiological state to undergo anaesthesia and surgery.

2. *Special preparation* is designed to modify and mitigate the effects upon the management of anaesthesia of any incidental pathology from which the patient is suffering.

Apparatus

Inhalational apparatus (Chapter 7) has two purposes:-

1. To deliver a gas mixture to the patient which includes sufficient oxygen to preserve life.

2. To deliver inhalation agents in an adequate but safe concentration.

Cessation of oxygen supply to the patient will cause permanent brain damage in four to eight minutes and will be followed by cardiac arrest[2]. Deliberate hypoxia was an important element in early nitrous oxide anaesthesia, but its use is not acceptable in modern anaesthetic practice; in fact, whenever possible, the concentration of oxygen should be greater than the 21% in air because the gradient between oxygen in the alveoli and in the arteries increases under anaesthesia[3]. The difference is marginal and of little physical significance to the fit subject under normal conditions; in fact many millions of anaesthetics have been given to patients using air (21% oxygen) alone as a carrier gas without harm,

[1] See also Chapter 8.

[2] 'Hypoxia' means lack of oxygen and 'anoxia' absence of oxygen, but the terms are often incorrectly used as synonyms.

[3] The reasons for this difference between the conscious and the anaesthetised state are complex. They include central depression of spontaneous respiration, reduction of cardiac output, differences in alveolar ventilation/blood flow relationships, an increase in the closing volume, and a fall in the functional residual capacity of the lung, possibly from a reduction in the resting tone of the diaphragm.

but most modern anaesthetists prefer an inspired oxygen concentration of at least 30% to increase the margin of safety. Oxygen concentrations over 30% are, of course, mandatory in certain conditions and circumstances — including cardiovascular disease, pregnancy, the elderly, patients with sickle cell anaemia, and at altitude.

The anaesthetist's principal duty is therefore to make certain that his apparatus is delivering an adequate concentration of oxygen to the patient. He must ensure that:

1. Oxygen is being supplied to the machine from the cylinder or pipeline outlet or the atmosphere.

2. The cylinder or pipeline is connected to the correct inlet on the machine without leaks. This is made easier by the modern pin non-interchangeable index system (Chapter 7).

3. The oxygen rotameter indicates an adequate flow in correct proportion to the nitrous oxide or other gas in use.

4. The total fresh gas flow is adequate to eliminate carbon dioxide from the particular breathing system in use, (Chapter 7).

5. The apparatus is connected to the patient without leaks.

Ventilators. It cannot be emphasised too strongly that a patient who has been paralysed with a muscle relaxant is dependent for his life on artificial intermittent positive pressure ventilation (IPPV) of his lungs, either manually by the anaesthetist or vicariously by a mechanical ventilator. A ventilator is not a substitute for the anaesthetist but merely a useful tool; it must be constantly supervised, never left unattended, and should have an alarm system to warn of disconnection leaks or excessive pressure.

Intravenous apparatus has other important functions besides providing a route for the administration of anaesthetic agents. It can be used to deliver antidotes and emergency drugs, and to infuse intravenous fluids to maintain blood volume and cardiac output in the face of haemorrhage and fluid loss.

Modern anaesthetists generally insist for safety on secure venous access before starting to anaesthetise a patient — exceptionally (in small children with difficult veins for example) this is achieved immediately after inhalation induction.

Emergency equipment must be on hand. This must include a powerful pharyngeal sucker (to protect the airway from the aspiration of regurgitated stomach contents), a cardiac defibrillator and electrocardiograph, and emergency drugs. A means of positive pressure ventilation with oxygen-enriched ambient air, such as a manual resuscitation bag or bellows, should be available also (Chapter 14).

The golden rule in failure or apparent malfunction of the anaesthetic apparatus or ventilator is to disconnect the offending device and use alternative equipment, — or even ventilate with your own expired gas blown directly into the tube or mouth.

The airway of the patient

All the oxygen in the world will be to no avail if it cannot be drawn into the patient's lungs down the patient's airway and taken by the circulation to his brain. The airway of the anaesthetised patient extends from his connection with the apparatus (either via an anaesthetic mask or through an endotracheal tube) to his alveolar membrane. Obstruction can, and does, occur anywhere in between. If it is complete and allowed to persist, the patient is as effectively deprived of oxygen as if the oxygen tap on the apparatus were turned off, and he will surely die.

Obstruction to the airway of the patient during anaesthesia sometimes occurs suddenly and demands prompt recognition, location and relief.

Corrugated tubing connecting the apparatus and the patient can become kinked and obstructed whether a mask or endotracheal tube is being used[4]. Obstruction to both inspiration and expiration can therefore occur if a circle type system is being employed. Obstruction to expiration can also be caused by compression or kinking of the tubing used to scavenge exhaled anaesthetic mixtures and conduct them to the exterior.

Obstruction from the tongue falling back. This is the commonest form of obstruction in the unconscious patient whether in the operating theatre, in the recovery room, or at a road accident. It is usually easily relievable, but at accidents it frequently kills. The treatment is to pull the jaw forward (Figure 6.1) with the patient lying on his back, and draw the point of the jaw towards the ceiling or sky. This manoeuvre may be performed simply by two fingers placed under the centre of the chin, although it may sometimes be easier to press the angles of the jaw forward with the thumbs. From this advice it is seen that if the point of the the jaw is conscientiously held forward during the entire administration, obstruction is avoided. The conventional grip for an anaesthetic mask uses two hands and includes the application of the index and middle fingers to the jaw, with the little finger hooked round the angle of the mandible if necessary; the

[4] A novel form of obstruction of connecting corrugated tubing was observed some years ago. A supervising anaesthetist was watching a medical student maintain an anaesthetic through the porthole in the operating theatre door. The patient was breathing adequately and the student, satisfied that all was well, sat down on the anaesthetist's stool to make himself comfortable. Immediately he sat down the reservoir bag ceased to move. The agitated student observing this stood up with the intention of examining the mask and valve in order to see what was wrong, whereupon the patient once again began to breathe adequately. The student, much relieved sat down once more, but immediately respiration ceased again. The student got up again and the patient started to breathe immediately. This cycle was repeated several times until the anaesthetist could bear it no longer, and stopped the student sitting on the corrugated tube.

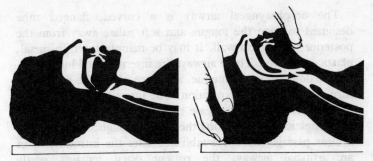

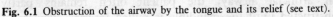

Fig. 6.1 Obstruction of the airway by the tongue and its relief (see text).

thumb and index finger push gently downwards to maintain a seal with the mask on the patient's face. With practice, in suitable patients, only one hand may be needed to hold the mask, thus freeing the other for record keeping, adjusting the anaesthetic apparatus or more personal activities.

It is surprising how often the simple action of drawing the jaw forward — and so pulling the tongue forward by its muscular attachments to the mandible — is successful in preventing what appears to be impending disaster. You may one day find yourself hurriedly called to the recovery room or ward to discover your last patient deeply cyanosed and under the energetic care of three nurses, the trio performing artificial respiration and administering oxygen with no effect. Often the only manoeuvre required is a firm forward tug on the patient's chin. Alternatively, if the patient is turned onto his side, gravity will almost always allow the jaw and tongue to be drawn away from the posterior wall of the pharynx and the airway will be cleared[5].

[5] Unconscious patients laid on their backs staring up to heaven, are closer to their Maker than they could possibly know. 'He who looks to heaven will soon be there.'

The oropharyngeal airway is a curved, flanged tube designed to keep the tongue and soft palate away from the posterior pharyngeal wall. It may be manufactured in metal, plastic or rubber. These airways are inserted, well lubricated, upside down over the tongue, and once inside the mouth are turned to their proper position. The insertion of such pieces of apparatus does not release the anaesthetist or nurse from the obligation of supporting the jaw. Although, in many cases a clear passage may be established after the introduction of an artificial airway, the patient often remains partly obstructed until the mandible is pulled forward. Beware of negroid and some asiatic races in whom the thick lips may shut over the flange of the airway and cause complete obstruction.

Occasionally the teeth are clenched so firmly that the insertion of an airway is impossible. This is a contingency likely during induction and at the end of a light anaesthetic; a length of cut endotracheal tube (No.7 or 8 for an adult) or a manufactured plastic or rubber nasopharyngeal airway may be passed through the nares and advanced to the hypopharynx; as soon as the tube passes the dorsum of the tongue, free breath sounds will be heard. The anaesthetist must not omit first to lubricate the tube, to take care in its passage through the nose, and to fasten a safety pin through its exposed end if it is not fitted with a flange[6]. The passage of tubes through the nose, though convenient on occasion, can easily cause severe haemorrhage.

Obstruction with saliva is less frequent with modern agents than with ether. Salivary secretion can be reduced by preme-

---

[6] Stories abound of patients returned to wards with nasal airways in situ. These may then be mistaken for a surgical drain and shortened an inch each day by the nursing staff. Routine postoperative visits by the anaesthetist would eliminate the problem before patients complain of difficulty in eating because of crumbs being blown out through the tube.

dication with atropine or glycopyrrolate and removed by suction.

Obstruction of the pharynx from active vomiting. This is unusual when patients for elective surgery have been properly starved, but occurs occasionally in patients who have disobeyed orders to abstain from food and drink, and in emergencies. Fortunately, in all but the most feeble patients, it occurs at a light stage of anaesthesia when active laryngeal reflexes are present. The patient should be turned on his side and the vomitus aspirated.

Obstruction from passive regurgitation is a dangerous complication. It occurs particularly after intravenous induction followed by a muscle relaxant before the trachea can be intubated. The consequences and the precautions which can be taken to avoid the disastrous soiling of the trachea by aspiration of the stomach contents are discussed in Chapter 11.

Obstruction from laryngeal spasm in the unintubated patient is more likely during induction, though it may arise at any time during the administration of anaesthesia or the recovery period. It can be either partial or complete.

The diagnosis of partial laryngeal spasm is made from the signs of obstruction plus a characteristic high pitched crowing from the larynx, (if the neck is touched lightly the vibration gives the sensation of handling a purring cat). The spasm, whether partial or complete, usually follows irritation of the larynx, by too rapid an increase in anaesthetic vapour, by blood, mucus or vomit, by a foreign body such as an airway, by endotracheal intubation attempted under too light anaesthesia, or by direct or reflex stimulation of the glottis due to the surgery if the patient is not intubated.

Any surgical manipulation may cause reflex partial, (or occasionally complete) laryngeal spasm if the anaesthesia is not sufficiently deep. Note that the depth of anaesthesia required is relative to the part handled, and that a plane of narcosis deep enough when the skin is cut may nevertheless allow spasm to follow such manoeuvres as handling the testis, the peritoneum, or the under surface of the diaphragm, or dilating the cervix or anus.

Hypoxic muscle goes into spasm, and the adductors of the vocal cords are no exception. Hence the 'vicious circle' — spasm of the larynx produces oxygen lack, which in turn increases the laryngeal spasm to augment the hypoxia. This circle must be broken swiftly, although in extremity most patients will take a final breath and an anaesthetic mask over the face may then deliver enough oxygen to permit survival, but this is not a solution to be relied on.

The intravenous barbiturates, particularly thiopentone (the most commonly used induction agent today), can predispose to spasm of the larynx. Spasm may occur when the induction is continued with inhalation anaesthesia administered in too high a concentration, even with the so-called non-irritant vapours, and may remain for some time. This danger has probably been overstressed in the past, but must be borne in mind. The respiratory tract of smokers and asthmatics is unduly sensitive and may go into bronchospasm or coughing in response to any form of mechanical irritation — including laryngoscopy and intubation.

Remember that the insertion of a pharyngeal airway immediately after induction with thiopentone may cause troublesome laryngeal spasm, and that tracheal tubes should never be passed under thiopentone anaesthesia alone. Note also that a dose of thiopentone may depress respiration to an extent that completely obscures the picture of obstruction by preventing respiratory efforts.

Obstruction of the upper respiratory tract from anatomical and pathological deformity. There may be maxillofacial, congenital, traumatic or pathological deformities of the oropharynx, or tumours in the lumen. Problems usually arise from the administration of a muscle relaxant before an attempt at intubation, rather than from obstruction in the spontaneously breathing patient. Patients with tumours or oedema of the larynx, or with a pathologically large tongue, may obstruct as soon as they are anaesthetised, particularly after intravenous induction, and the greatest care is needed. Inhalation induction or awake intubation may be necessary.

Obstruction after tracheal intubation. Although induction with an intravenous agent, muscular paralysis with a neuro-muscular blocking relaxant, and rapid intubation avoid many of the complications associated with obstruction of the upper airway mentioned above, obstruction can still occur.

Some schools of anaesthesia, particularly those involved with the care of children, regard tracheal intubation as mandatory for safety's sake; but their patients may suffer other morbid effects as sore throat and laryngeal oedema.

Obstruction of the lumen of the tracheal tube or the adaptors which connect it to the anaesthetic system (the catheter mount and suction union), may occur in several ways. The catheter mount can become twisted, or the tube kinked at the teeth or in the back of the pharynx, the bevel of the tube may abut against the wall of the trachea when the neck is twisted or the head extended, or the lumen of the tube may be blocked by a foreign body or with sputum or blood. Suction will solve the latter problem, repositioning of the tube the others. Another danger is the introduction of a long endotracheal tube into the right bronchus, making the left lung inoperative and causing hypoxia.

Bronchospasm may occur whether the patient is intubated or not. It may also be part of an anaphylactic response to a drug (see Chapter 13).

Respiration and ventilation

Even if there is no physical obstruction of the airway, oxygen is useless to the patient unless it can be drawn or pushed into the lungs and the waste product, carbon dioxide, eliminated.

It is essential to monitor spontaneous respiration, which may be centrally depressed by many of the drugs used in anaesthesia. The importance of supervising mechanical ventilators has already been stressed. Anaesthetists should get into the habit of watching the chest move rather than observing the movements of the bag or bellows, which may become disconnected from the patient.

The circulation

Oxygen reaching the alveoli must diffuse into the blood across the alveolar membrane, bind to haemoglobin in the red cell, and then be circulated to the brain. Careful preoperative treatment of cardiac disease and restoration of blood volume when required are essential.

Some agents depress cardiac output and/or cause cardiac irregularities. These effects are discussed in the appropriate chapters. Safety demands careful monitoring of blood pressure, pulse rate, and cardiac rhythm. Most anaesthetists now regard the electrocardiograph (ECG) as mandatory throughout all cases.

Blood volume must be maintained. Losses during anaesthesia must be assessed and replaced as appropriate.

Explosions and fires

Cyclopropane, a highly explosive anaesthetic gas, is rarely used today because of its flammability. Operating theatre construction is simpler and cheaper if explosive agents are forbidden and expensive precautions like antistatic floors are avoided. This attitude to operating theatre construction is already commonplace in North America and is likely to spread to the United Kingdom. The absence of antistatic floors contraindicates the use of ether. This is a pity, as it is arguably the safest inhalational agent, and certainly the cheapest and most readily available worldwide. It also has many advantages in elderly and hypovolaemic patients. It is probably still the most commonly used anaesthetic in the more isolated rural areas of less developed countries. The recommendation in Britain is that ether should not be used when the cautery or other naked source of ignition is used, nor without antistatic precautions which are fortunately still provided in the United Kingdom. Any anaesthetist who uses ether while the cautery is in use does so on his own responsibility. What are the facts however? Ether/air mixtures are less likely to ignite and rarely explode. The risk is therefore less than when ether/oxygen or ether/nitrous oxide/oxygen mixtures are used as these are dangerously explosive. Ether/air drawover anaesthesia (Chapter 7) administered by an occasional anaesthetist in a developing country may be less hazardous than the use of a more potent nonflammable agent with which he is not familiar. It is some comfort to remember that no explosion has ever been reported when ether has been given with air as the carrier gas[7], and ether in oxygen is so diluted with air 30 cm from the expiratory valve or the source of a leak that ignition by an electric spark is not possible; also ether is heavier than air and falls to the floor away from the operating site. With common sense and care ether *can* be given while cautery is in use on the abdomen, but it is a different matter if the surgeon larks about with cautery or heated bulbs in the mouth!

The danger from electric sparks without antistatic precautions and floors is more serious in a hot dry country, particularly if building regulations are not stringent. The use of a large damp linen sheet covering the floor of the operating area, and wetting the inside of antistatic tubing before use

[7] A well known academic anaesthetist was in the habit of proving the point by holding a match to the face of baboons whom he had anaesthetised with open ether.

goes some way to overcoming this difficulty in primitive conditions. The separate danger of fire from someone dropping a bottle of ether near electric apparatus which is not sparkproof should be borne in mind.

Operating theatre health hazards

Concern has been shown in recent years about the particular health hazards confronting personnel working in operating theatres. These include the dangers of exposure to radiation and infection especially with serum B hepatitis from symptomless carriers, and lately the risk of acquiring autoimmune deficiency syndrome (AIDS). Reasonable protective and decontamination measures should be taken.

Pollution from waste anaesthetic gas mixtures has caused concern over increased abortion risk and possible mutagenic dangers. There is statistical evidence that women working in operating theatres have an increased abortion risk, but not of fetal abnormality. This may not be directly the result of inhalation of trace amounts of anaesthetics. As a wise precaution, most British operating theatres have introduced passive or active scavenging systems; as a possible consequence, many anaesthetists believe themselves to be less tired at the end of the day.

Addiction. Anaesthetists belong to one of the few medical disciplines who directly administer drugs as well as prescribe them. They must always guard against misuse themselves and amongst their colleagues. Nitrous oxide, volatile agents, narcotics, and often drugs of addiction are temptingly readily available.

7

Apparatus

'And now I see with eye serene the very pulse of the machine'
Perfect Woman   William Wordsworth (1770–1850).

Like Wordsworth, anaesthetists are discriminating and well informed, and seek good design and efficiency when they choose their machines.

The administration of anaesthesia

Modern anaesthesia requires provision for:
1. the delivery of oxygen to the patient
2. the administraton of gaseous and/or volatile anaesthetic agents
3. the elimination of carbon dioxide
4. controlled ventilation
5. the monitoring of cardiac, pulmonary and other body functions and the performance of apparatus
6. intravenous injection and infusion
7. intramuscular and subcutaneous injection
8. the administration of local anaesthetics.

Anaesthetic machines

The term 'anaesthetic machine' is traditional for an apparatus which delivers oxygen and gaseous and/or volatile agents.

51

There are two types which will provide all the requirements for modern inhalational anaesthesia. These are the 'continuous flow' and 'drawover' machines. A third type, 'demand flow' apparatus, was designed for spontaneous respiration but not for controlled ventilation and is fast becoming obsolete.

Continuous flow anaesthetic machines

The generic name which the British anaesthetist gives to his continuous flow apparatus is the 'Boyle machine', after H. E. Gaskin Boyle (1875–1941), Consultant Anaesthetist to St Bartholomew's Hospital, London, who developed and popularised the continuous flow technique shortly after World War I.[1]

The modern continuous flow anaesthetic machine is a complicated device as technically different from the original Boyle machines as the modern car from the original Model T Ford. The main components are:-

1. A source of supply for compressed anaesthetic gases (cylinders and/or a piped supply).
2. Reducing valves
3. Flow restrictors
4. Flow meters (rotameters)
5. Vaporisers
6. Gas delivery systems ensuring the elimination of carbon dioxide
7. Ventilators
8. Warning and safety devices
9. Scavenging systems.

[1] The original Boyle machine was derived from that introduced by the American, J. T. Gwathmey (1863–1944), and also owed much to an apparatus designed by Geoffrey Marshall (1886–1983) of Guy's Hospital, London, which was used in France by the British Expeditionary Force in World War I.

The supply of anaesthetic gases

Oxygen is usually stored centrally as a liquid in most British hospitals and piped to the operating theatre suite and elsewhere. Liquid oxygen is pumped from a lorry into a thermally insulated storage tank where it is kept at a pressure of 10.5 bar and a temperature between -175 and $-150°C$. Reserve cylinders of compressed gaseous oxygen at 126 bar are kept on each anaesthetic machine.

Nitrous oxide is usually stored under pressure as a liquid in banks of large cylinders at 50 kPa with smaller cylinders in reserve on each anaesthetic machine.

Carbon dioxide (CO_2) is used as a respiratory stimulant in certain anaesthetic techniques. It is contained in small cylinders at 50 kPa mounted on the anaesthetic machine. Some British anaesthetists, and nearly all anaesthesiologists in the USA regard the permanent presence of a CO_2 cylinder on the machine as potentially dangerous because the gas may be accidentally introduced into the anaesthetic circuit; at the very least the CO_2 cylinder should be turned off when not actually in use.

Compressed air — stored in cylinders at 137 kPa — is provided for addition to the carrier gas mixture on the modern continuous flow machines, or may be piped to the operating theatre.

Cylinders (or 'tanks' in the USA) are colour coded (Table 7.1) and attached to the apparatus by a metal yoke with pins which fit only the holes in the cylinder heads of one particular gas. This is the 'pin-index' system, which prevents the wrong cylinder being fixed to the wrong yoke. A special washer (a Bodok seal) between the yoke and the cylinder head ensures a gas-tight fit.

If piped gases are not used, labels indicate which of the pair of cylinders for each gas is 'in use' or 'full' for nitrous oxide and oxygen. There is a single cylinder of carbon dioxide but

Table 7.1 Gas cylinders commonly used in anaesthesia in the United Kingdom

Gas	Symbol	Cylinder colour	Physical State	Pressure when full (Bar*)
Oxygen	O_2	Black with white shoulder	Gas	136
Nitrous oxide	N_2O	French blue	Liquid	50
Premixed 50 % O_2 50% N_2O	O_2/N_2O	French blue with white shoulder	Gas (above $-70°C$)	47
Carbon dioxide	CO_2	Grey	Gas	137
Air	–	Grey with white and black shoulders	Gas	137
Cyclopropane	C_3H_6	Orange	Liquid	5

* 1 Bar = kilo Pascals (kPa × 100)
The colour codes used in the United Kingdom are those authorised by International agreement. Other countries do not necessarily conform, particularly in the matter of identifying oxygen, which is, for example, in green cylinders in the USA.

two each of oxygen and nitrous oxide. An empty cylinder should always be changed as soon as possible, and the anaesthetist must ensure that there is a full reserve cylinder. Empty cylinders must be stored separately from the full ones. Full cylinders have the orifice on the head covered by a plastic seal; this must be removed before the cylinder is fitted to the apparatus.

Reducing valves are fitted at the liquid oxygen tank or the cylinder bank to reduce the pressure delivered to the machine to 4 kPa. The pipelines lead to a colour-coded gas point and Schraeder quick release valves, and thence by colour-coded flexible hoses to the anaesthetic machine without further pressure reduction. Reducing valves also form an integral part of the machine, to reduce the pressure in the locally mounted cylinders to 4 kPa.

The valves are not interchangeable from one gas to another.

A spring loaded diaphragm counteracts the cylinder pressure, and must be promptly replaced if faulty or noisy. The valves carry a gauge informing the anaesthetist of the pressure of gas remaining in the cylinder. The pressure of the oxygen is directly related to the amount of gas, but as nitrous oxide is normally liquid in the cylinder, the reading on the gauge remains high until it is all in gaseous form and then the reading gradually goes down.

Flow restrictors (constrictions in the metal pipe between the pipeline attachment or the reducing valve and the flowmeters) smooth out the surges which might follow changes in pressure in the connecting pipes from alterations in the flow of gases.

Needle valves, activated by screw control knobs are used by the anaesthetist to adjust the gas flow to the flowmeters. A further drop in pressure occurs across the valves.

Flowmeters measure the flow of each gas to the patient and pass the gases into a common conduit. The commonest type of flowmeter on anaesthetic machines today is the accurate 'rotameter', in which duralumin bobbins spin in the gas flow clear of the walls of a tapered glass tube, so avoiding the effects of friction. These bobbins are read from their flat tops, and the rotameter is calibrated in 100 ml per minute and/or in litres per minute.

Vaporisers. The mixed gases now pass into the entry port of a vaporiser. If the vaporiser is turned off the flow of gas passes straight through a bypass duct. When a dial or lever is turned, the flow is partially diverted into the vaporising chamber to pick up volatile anaesthetic vapour. The amount delivered is dependent on the flow diverted, the design of the vaporiser, and the provision for compensation for falls in temperature because of the vaporisation of the agents.

Accurate vaporisers, each for a single agent, became essential in continuous flow machines when the highly potent volatile agent halothane (Fluothane)® was introduced in the nineteen fifties. Those most commonly used have thermostatic devices which compensate for temperature changes and are accurate over a wide range of flow rates.

Manufacturers and international standard authorities now encourage the use of only a single agent and vaporiser at a time to avoid contamination of one agent by another.

Lock-on devices allow for easy exchange of vaporisers and aid routine servicing and recalibration of individual vaporisers, which should be done at least once each year.

An alternative method of providing an accurate percentage of volatile agent in the mixture, less popular in the United Kingdom than in the USA, is a device like the 'copper kettle'. This adds a known flow rate of saturated vapour in oxygen to the main stream from a separate rotameter.

The anaesthetic mixture passes from the vaporiser through another flow restrictor (to prevent the effect of back pressure if controlled ventilation is employed) into the gas delivery system (see below).

Formerly simple 'glass jar' vaporisers, such as the Boyle's bottle, were used[2]. The concentrations delivered by such devices diminish as the vaporising liquid evaporates and cools, and vary with the extent of the surface area of the liquid exposed to the gas flow, the rate of gas flow, the position of the bypass lever, and in with the Boyle's bottle, of the plunger and hood which directed the flow of gases close to, or even bubbled it below the surface of the volatile agent. The exact concentration of vapour delivered was unpredictable and, though wide variations are acceptable when anaesthetics of low potency such as ether are used, they became dangerous when powerful new agents as halothane were available. The Goldman vaporiser was designed for halothane and

[2] Apart from the advantage of being transparent, glass is almost the worst possible material for use as a vaporising chamber. It conducts a negligible amount of heat from the outside, and therefore the temperature of the liquid agent and the concentration of the vapour fall rapidly at the start of the anaesthetic.

limited the maximum concentration to a safe level by utilising a small glass container.

Continuous gas delivery system

The elimination of carbon dioxide (CO_2) from continuous flow systems can be achieved in two ways:

1. A high flow system is used in which fresh gases flush CO_2 out of the system during the expiratory pause.

2. A circle system is employed in which the CO_2 is absorbed by soda lime[3]; in practice the relief valve of the circle system is often left partly opened and some of the CO_2 is absorbed and some flushed out.

Gas delivery systems employing high continuous gas flows but no soda lime absorbtion

These systems are confusingly sometimes called 'semi-open' and sometimes 'semiclosed' in British textbooks. Both terms are best avoided especially as they are used about closed systems by the Americans. It is better to use the names of the various originators (like Magill, Bain, Ayre, and Jackson Rees), or the well known alphabetical classification of Mapleson. The Mapleson B and C systems are rarely used and can be forgotten. Hooded valves can be fitted to most of these systems to adapt them for the scavenging of pollutant anaesthetic mixtures (Chapter 6).

Magill (Mapleson A) system or 'attachment' is probably the most frequently used gas delivery system in the United

---

[3] Soda lime is a granular mixture of 90% calcium hydroxide and 5% sodium bihydroxide with silicates which prevent powder formation. The CO_2 combines with the hydroxides to form carbonates. Soda lime often contains an indicator which changes colour as the hydroxides are neutralised.

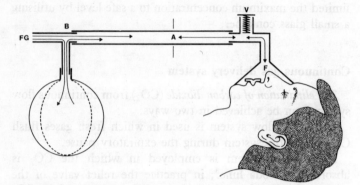

Fig. 7.1 The Magill, or Mapleson A breathing system (see text).
F = Apparatus dead space V = Expiratory valve FG = Fresh gas
B = Reservoir bag and bag mount AV = Patient's exhaled dead space gas

Kingdom for the spontaneously respiring patient.[4]

The device (Figure 7.1) consists of a two litre bag on a T-shaped mount (B) at the end nearest the machine, a one metre length of low resistance, wide bore, corrugated tubing (diameter about 30 mm) and a spring loaded low resistance (V) Heidbrink (or 'pop-off') valve next to the face mask (F).

Let us assume that the apparatus dead space at (F) between the mouth and the valve is negligible, and an adult patient is about to exhale after inspiring a tidal volume of approximately 600 ml. The reservoir bag will then be partly but not completely deflated after the inspiration. The patient begins to breathe out. The first portion of his exhaled gases, (say one third or 200 ml), will not escape through the valve (V) because it is held closed by the spring. It will, however,

---

[4] The Lack system is a variant of the Magill (Mapleson A) which conducts the gases from the patient end of the system via a coaxial inner tube to a valve placed remotely from the face of the patient which can be capped for scavenging. It is thus the reverse of the Bain system described later in which the fresh gases are delivered via the inner coaxial tube.

overcome the continuous fresh gas (FG) flow from the machine, which will be diverted into the reservoir bag at (B) and come to occupy the section of corrugated tubing between (V) and the point A. There will be little CO_2 in the first portion of exhaled gases, which is dead space gas from the mouth and pharynx. This has not taken part in the gaseous exchange of respiration.

The reservoir bag has now expanded sufficiently to cause a rise in tension in the system, the valve (V) opens and the remaining two thirds of the exhalation (approximately 400 ml) containing near alveolar gas with a high concentration of CO_2 passes out. During the expiratory pause of about one second which follows a normal exhalation, fresh gases from the apparatus will flow towards (V) and force out the small quantity of gas with a high concentration of CO_2 in the vicinity of the valve. Inspiration follows. The valve (V) closes and the patient inspires an aliquot of CO_2-free dead space gas between (V) and A which he exhaled, plus fresh gases from the machine and from the reservoir bag.

The Magill (Mapleson A) system functions efficiently to eliminate CO_2 if the patient is breathing spontaneously and the volume delivered by the machine is about 70% of the patient's minute volume (between 4 and 5 l/min in an adult patient with a tidal volume of 600 ml), but it is unusual for the system to be used with a flow as low as 5 l/min. A flow of 2.5 l/min of oxygen plus 5 l/min of N_2O (total 7.5 litres/min) gives the 33% oxygen mixture acceptable to most anaesthetists.

The Magill system is rarely used for controlled ventilation, except briefly in the anaesthetic room when flows of 9 l/min or more are used to flush out the CO_2. If it is used for a long period for controlled ventilation the valve must be tightened for inspiration and slackened for the expiratory phase. If the patient is intubated, the Heidbrink valve may be closed, the bung in the suction port on the tracheal tube connector

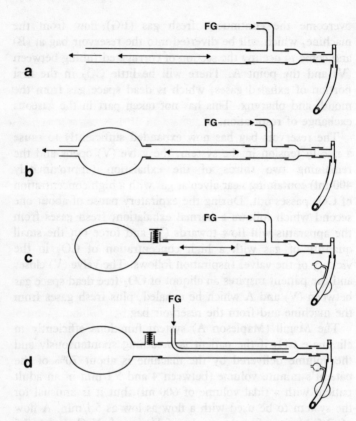

Fig. 7.2 T-Piece breathing systems.
(a) Ayres T-piece (Mapleson E) (b) Jackson Rees' modification of Ayres T-piece (Mapleson F) (c) The Mapleson D breathing system. (d) The Bain breathing system (Coaxial Mapleson D) FG = Fresh gas

removed, and the finger used to close it intermittently each time the bag is squeezed.

Ayre's T-piece (Mapleson E system) consists of a T-piece without valves with a long expiratory limb (Figure 7.2a). It was originally designed for cleft palate surgery in spontaneously respiring infants and was popular for paediatric anaesthesia. It has a low resistance as it does not have valves and solves the difficulty with apparatus dead space which is important for the smaller patient. Ayre's T-piece is shown with a tracheal tube in Figure 7.2a. The use of a tube will reduce dead space further. The end expired CO_2 will be maximal near the gas inlet at the end of the expiratory phase. The device relies on the fresh gas flow (FG) during the expiratory pause to flush out the CO_2 and fill the expiratory limb with fresh gases ready for inspiration. It has been calculated that a fresh gas flow of twice the minute volume is required (3 l/min for a small infant, 8 l/min for a 4-year-old child). Theoretically there is no limit to the length of the expiratory limb, but if it is too long resistance increases; if it is too short the anaesthetic is diluted with air.

Jackson Rees modification of Ayre's T-piece is the addition of an open-ended small rubber bag to the expiratory limb (Fig. 7.2b). The device is universally used for controlled ventilation in small children. The anaesthetist should control the leak between his fourth and fifth fingers and squeeze the bag one handed to ventilate the lungs; this ensures that he can feel changes in lung compliance, disconnexions, and the return of spontaneous breathing efforts, etc.

The Bain system

The Bain system (Fig. 7.2d)[5] is in fact, an elegant coaxial (Mapleson D system (Fig. 7.2c) with the gas delivery tube inside the lumen of the expiratory limb. The Bain system is

[5] The system now classified as the coaxial Mapleson D and popularised by Bain and Spoerel was used by Professor (now Sir) Robert Macintosh of Oxford during experiments to test life jackets during World War II. Dr (later Professor) E. A. Pask was himself anaesthetised and then immersed with his head under water in a swimming pool. It must be the only occasion in which the author of a Cambridge MD thesis was himself unconscious at the time of the experiments which were its subject.

particularly valuable for the management of operations on the head and neck because the valve is at the proximal end of the system under the control of the anaesthetist. There has been much controversy over the flow required to eliminate CO_2 when using the Bain system for spontaneously respiring adults. The system obviously resembles the Ayre's T-piece (Fig. 7.2a) and some anaesthetists insist that flows of over twice the minute volume are required in the adult (perhaps 15 l/minute or more). The original paper by Bain & Spoerel (1972) demonstrated that the system works satisfactorily in practice with flows of 7.5 l/min for adults and 5.5 l/min *all* others (including small children). The flow requirement is thus like the Ayre's T-piece and Jackson Rees systems — over twice the minute volume for small children but only 25% to 50% greater than the minute volume in adults. Adults breathe more slowly than small children and thus there is more time for the CO_2 to be flushed out in each cycle in the longer expiratory pause. The system is efficient for controlled ventilation with flows of 70 to 100 ml/kg body weight.

Continuous flow gas delivery system employing soda lime absorption

Removing expired carbon dioxide with soda lime, rather than flushing it out with high flows of gases, was introduced by Waters[6] about 1920 with a simple valveless 'to and fro' apparatus (Fig. 7.3). The more sophisticated valved, one way, circle absorption system (Fig. 7.4) was initiated by Brian Sword (1889–1956) of New Haven, Connecticut in 1926.

Advantages. These systems were invented for economy. The patient rebreathes the unused expired oxygen and anaesthetic mixture to a greater or lesser extent; theoretically all that needs to be added to a completely closed circle is a basal

[6] Ralph Milton Waters (1883–1979) became the first Professor of Anaesthesia when he was elected by the University of Winsconsin in 1933.

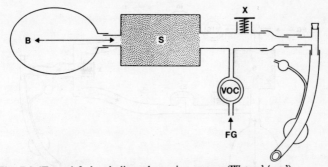

Fig. 7.3 'To and fro' soda lime absorption system (Waters' 'can').
B = Reservoir bag   S = Soda lime canister   FG = Fresh gas
VOC = Vaporiser outside the system   X = 'pop-off' valve   A vaporiser in
the VOC position may be a high resistence continuous flow vaporiser but
the concentration inside the system is unpredictable unless a relatively
high flow is used (see text).

requirement of oxygen (about 250 ml/min for an adult) to
replace that metabolised and additional inhalational anaesthetic agent. Absorption systems increased in popularity after
the introduction of the effective, but expensive and explosive,
gaseous agent cyclopropane in the early 1930s. Absorption
systems remained popular in the USA and in continental
Europe but not in Britain even after the decline of cyclopropane. Interest has revived again in the United Kingdom since
closed rebreathing systems avoid atmospheric pollution and
save money with use of expensive volatile agents like halothane, enflurane and isoflurane.[7] Added advantages of
rebreathing systems are the retention of body heat and self-
humidification of the anaesthetic mixture.

[7] It is an interesting fact of social economics that United States
anesthesiologists, who were financed by personal or delegated departmental
budgeting, remained interested in the economics of anaesthesia and in
rebreathing, while British anaesthetists, under the umbrella of the all
provident British National Health Service, preferred the more profligate
high flow systems. One of the authors was very unpopular with his
American Chief when he introduced the 'wasteful' high flow Magill
(Mapleson A) circuit to the University of Michigan Hospital in 1956.

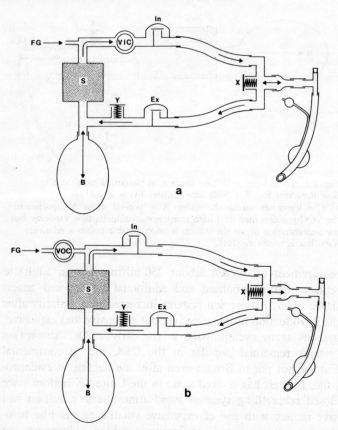

Fig. 7.4 Circle soda lime absorption systems.
FG = Fresh gas S = Soda lime canister B = Reservoir bag
In = Inspiratory valve Ex = Expiratory valve VIC = Vaporiser in 'circuit'
VOC = Vaporiser outside 'circuit' X and Y = Alternative positions for
the 'pop-off' valves.   Position X is best for spontaneous respiration,
position Y for controlled ventilation. (**a**) A low resistance vaporiser must
be used in the circuit (VIC). In the absence of devices for monitoring the
concentrations of the anaesthetic mixture it is best if it is relatively
inefficient for spontaneous respiration — so that when respiration is
depressed by the volatile agent a lower concentration is vaporised.
(**b**) A high resistance vaporiser may be used outside the 'circuit'. See text
for discussion of the use of circle absorption systems.

Disadvantages. The main disadvantage of rebreathing systems is that the composition of the inhaled anaesthetic mixture is not shown by the rotameter bobbins and vaporiser dials. The concentrations in an absorption system must either be crudely estimated by observing the patient's physical signs and kept safe by rule of thumb, learned with experience, or monitored by expensive electronic analysers to estimate the composition of the anaesthetic mixture. Safe use of a circle system may, therefore, be a false economy when the initial capital cost and subsequent expense of maintenance of the soda lime, its cannister and monitoring systems are added.

Rebreathing systems can either be used completely 'closed', employing only basal flow, or, more easily by the 'low flow' (American 'semiclosed') method in which more than the basal flow is given and the excess is vented by a 'pop-off' valve. The greater the gas flow, the greater the predictability of the inspired mixtures, but the less the economy of the system and the greater the risk of blowing dust from the soda lime into the patient's lungs, particularly with the 'to and fro' system. A 'low flow' circle system, after an initial wash-out with a flow of 7 l/min for the adult, will retain a reasonably predictable steady state at oxygen 1/min, nitrous oxide 2/min, and volatile anaesthetic at the concentration shown with the vaporiser outside the 'circuit' (VOC) and the 'pop-off' valve open (Figs. 7.3 and 7.4).

Draw-over anaesthetic apparatus

The principle of draw-over anaesthetic apparatus (Fig. 7.5) differs from the more common continuous flow machines. Atmospheric air is drawn into the vaporiser either by the patient's spontaneous breathing or by a bellows or self-expanding bag (a hand resuscitator used in cases of respiratory arrest). One way valves ensure that the anaesthetic mixture moves only into the patient's lungs, and out into the

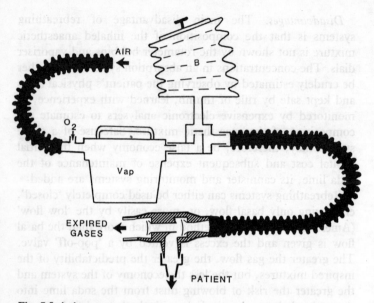

Fig. 7.5 A draw-over system.
Air is inspired into the corrugated reservoir tube and may be enriched
with oxygen at O_2. Vap = Low resistance vaporiser B = Bellows
surmounting an inspiratory valve. The valve illustrated (not to scale) is the
AMBU E1 anaesthetic valve which can operate for spontaneous respiration
or controlled ventilation without adjustment.

atmosphere (either directly or through a scavenging system)
during exhalation. The dual purpose expiratory valve (usually
the AMBU E1 or the Ruben valve) enables the patient to
breathe spontaneously or to have his ventilation controlled
without an adjustment having to be made between the use of
these modes.

The draw-over apparatus thus has everything required for
the administration of modern inhalational anaesthesia — a
means of delivering oxygen (in this case in ambient air) to the
patient, a calibrated vaporiser for delivering a volatile agent,

a means of eliminating expired carbon dioxide (the one-way valve system), and provision for controlled ventilation.

Draw-over systems used after intravenous anaesthetic agents, and as necessary with neuromuscular blocking agents, local anaesthesia and oxygen enrichment of the ambient air, are suitable for the administration of any modern general anaesthetic technique for any operation.

Draw-over systems, being portable and not dependent on compressed medical gases[8], are particularly valuable for use in the deprived rural areas of developing countries, and in battle or civil disaster conditions. If safe economical anaesthesia is needed for use by the anaesthetists in developing countries, ether in air is cheap, effective and safe — especially if used in minimal quantities with a muscle relaxant technique and controlled ventilation.

In battle or disaster conditions flammable ether must be avoided, economy is less important and the anaesthetists are usually specialists accustomed to using more potent volatile agents. The value of draw-over techniques was again demonstrated in the Falkland Islands campaign of 1983 using an air/oxygen and trichloroethylene and halothane technique.

---

[8] Ambient air will suffice as a carrier gas in most circumstances and oxygen concentrators are devices designed to absorb nitrogen from air leaving 95% oxygen which can be used to supplement ambient air for anaesthesia or oxygen therapy, thus avoiding the need for compressed gases in cylinders.

8

Anaesthesia for the fit patient

'The normal is what you find but rarely. The normal is an ideal.'

The Summing Up   Somerset Maugham (1874–1965)

Fortunately most surgical patients are fit apart from the condition which requires them to have an operation and anaesthetic. The anaesthetist is obliged to ensure that the patient is not harmed in any way, since he will remove the patient's ability to protect himself, and that the perioperative period is made as comfortable as possible. 'In somno securitas', (the motto of the Association of Anaesthetists of Great Britain and Ireland) summarises this tersely but accurately. This chapter outlines the proper conduct of a general anaesthetic for a fit adult undergoing elective surgery — the commonest task for the anaesthetist.

The anatomy of the anaesthetic

There are six stages in the management of the care of a patient in the perioperative period — assessment, preparation, premedication, anaesthesia, recovery, and aftercare.

The assessment

The American Society of Anesthesiologists (ASA) categories

Table 8.1   American Society of Anesthesiologists (ASA) Physical Status Categories (This risk classification is widely accepted internationally.)

ASA 1	A normal healthy patient with a localised condition requiring surgery.
ASA 2	A patient with a mild, or well controlled, systemic condition. e.g. mild hypertension, well controlled diabetes, old age.
ASA 3	A patient with severe systemic condition limiting life style. e.g. angina, a recent myocardial failure.
ASA 4	A patient with a severe systemic condition threatening life. e.g. advanced cardiac, pulmonary or renal disease.
ASA 5	A moribund patient not expected to survive 24 hours with or without operation. This category may include a previously fit patient with, for example, uncontrollable haemorrhage, as well as an elderly patient with a terminal disease.
E	This letter is placed before the numerical classification if the operation is an emergency.

Anesthesiology 1970; *33*: 130

give a useful overall assessment of anaesthetic risk (Table 8.1) physical status, which is universally accepted. In this chapter we are concerned with ASA categories 1 and 2.

The operating list. The anaesthetist's first sign of what he is to anaesthetise is usually the operating list, — often presented inconveniently late in the day after the surgical teams have organized their operating schedule. The operating list itself will give some clues (for instance, the patient's age and the proposed operation) which may warn that the case may not be straightforward. The name of the surgeon who is to operate and the time that the list is expected to start also provide important information for the anaesthetist, who must organize preoperative preparation and premedication and plan how to tackle the problems.

Armed with his own copy of the list the anaesthetist should go to the ward with the intention of making the patient as ready for surgery as possible within the time available.

The house surgeon's preoperative history and examination are really to ensure that the correct operation is scheduled and any necessary investigations prior to surgery are initiated, and only incidentally to assess the patient's fitness for anaesthesia, but the house surgeon's initial assessment is nonetheless useful.

If he is not well known in the particular ward, the anaesthetist should introduce himself to the nursing staff, tell them which patient he has come to see, and ask for any relevant information about the patient's condition, (for instance if the patient is deaf it is prudent to obtain a side-room to spare the others hearing your communicating by shouting).

The notes should then be read. The particular points to look for are:

1. Any history of previous anaesthetics. Note should be taken of the techniques and agents used, the type and size of tracheal tube, the site of infusion, the effect of premedication, airway difficulties, adverse reactions and any problems during recovery. The interval from any previous operation is important, because of the problems of repeated anaesthesia (see Ch. 12).
2. The present surgical condition requiring operation, and its specific site.
3. The state of patient's health as assessed by the surgical firm or by others.
4. Past history of medical disorders.
5. Any significant family or social history.
6. The medication which the patient is receiving.

Meeting the patient. After reading the notes, enquiring of the nurses and gaining all available information, the anaesthetist can approach the patient prepared to discuss the anaesthetic. The anaesthetist must never forget that he has the awesome responsibility of keeping the patient alive during surgery and that he is probably the only member of the surgical team who may be perceived by the patient to be unlikely to inflict stress and pain. It will be important to the patient that he feels that the anaesthetist — the last person he sees before losing consciousness — is actually concerned about him.

The anaesthetist should introduce himself, shake hands and sit down so that the patient can talk comfortably. The anaesthetist should explain that he intends to provide the most appropriate form of anaesthesia, and that it is therefore important to ask a few more questions and make any necessary examination. This may appear unnecessary to the patient as the house surgeon has already covered the ground, but patients are resigned to giving a history.

If the patient can answer 'No' to all the following, he can probably be regarded as fit. If the response is 'Yes' postponement of elective surgery and further investigation or modification of the anaesthetic technique may be required.

1. *Do you have a cold, cough or sore throat?* Patients with acute upper respiratory infections should have elective surgery postponed — at best they feel lousy in the postoperative period; at worst, they develop serious postoperative chest infection.

2. *Do you get short of breath on climbing one flight of stairs?* A positive answer may indicate that the patient is merely overweight, or that the patient has a serious cardiopulmonary condition requiring further investigation and treatment.

3. *Do you have to be propped up in bed with more than two pillows to sleep properly?* If the answer is 'Yes' the patient may have serious cardiopulmonary disease, which requires investigation. Or he may suffer from reflux oesophagitis, for which treatment with an H_2 histamine receptor blocker will be indicated (e.g. rantidine 150 mg every eight hours), and intubation performed with special precautions to separate the respiratory and gastrointestinal tracts to avoid aspiration damage.

4. *Do your ankles swell?* Bilateral swelling of the ankles, particularly on wakening in the morning may indicate congestive cardiac failure. Unilateral swelling suggests localised venous congestion and possible thrombosis. Anticoagulation measures ranging from the wearing of supportive stockings to the use of anticoagulants such as heparin may then be indicated.

5. *Do you get chest pain?* Chest pain must never be ignored. The presence of coronary ischaemia is a serious hazard. Tachycardia, or a lowered blood pressure may precipitate actual myocardial infarction. A patient with exertional chest pain certainly should not be allowed to undergo elective surgery without further investigation and treatment.

6. *Do you have palpitations?* Many people have palpitations in times of stress but their presence may indicate significant disease. If the patient has palpitations which are regular he may be suffering from anxiety, or drug abuse, or simply have a poor exercise tolerance. Irregular palpitations indicate either atrial fibrillation or ventricular ectopics caused by myocardial weakness. Any patient with a cardiac irregularity is likely to develop a worse dysrhythmia under anaesthesia. Such patients should be referred to a cardiologist in the hope of improvement before elective surgery is undertaken.

7. *Have you or close relatives had problems with anaesthesia?* Few patients are told if there have been transient anaesthetic complications, but the patient will probably have been warned to inform future anaesthetists if he has suffered an anaphylactic response or is hypersensitive to certain agents, such as induction agents or muscle relaxants. The patient will know if there were difficulties with venepuncture or if he had postoperative nausea and vomiting, but possibly not if there were intubation problems or spikes of postoperative pyrexia indicating the

possibility of halothane related hepatitis. Information about these conditions may be obtained from the patient's previous notes. Very occasionally there may be a startling history of family deaths or morbidity under anaesthesia which may indicate a familial tendency to the dangerous condition of malignant hyperpyrexia. Another example is prolonged apnoea following succinylcholine due to the inherited presence of abnormal plasma cholinesterase.

8. *Have you had scarlet fever, diphtheria or rheumatic fever?* Scarlet fever and diphtheria may result in cardiac conduction defects. Rheumatic fever may leave a legacy of valvular heart disease necessitating prophylactic antibiotic therapy, to prevent endocarditis from a shower of bacteria in the blood released by surgery.

9. *Are you being treated for hypertension, diabetes, or epilepsy?* These chronic conditions may normally be well controlled but the patient may have failed to take his medication in the preoperative period. Some anaesthetic drugs, including enflurane and methohexitone may precipitate convulsions.

10. *Are you taking any drugs or medication?* The medicines indicate that the patient has a medical condition recognised by someone else, which is serious enough to warrant treatment. The drugs which particularly concern anaesthetists are those which alter the effects of the anaesthetic either by interfering with drug metabolism, as described above, or by exaggerating the effects of the anaesthetic drugs. Any central nervous system depressant may increase the effect on the hypnotic and analgesic drugs given during anaesthesia. Drug interactions will be discussed later. The drugs concerned range from the socially-indicated contraceptive pill, to steroids or insulin, which if withheld, could be fatal.

11. *Are you allergic to anything?* The 'allergies' which a patient

may have range from major, life threating anaphylaxis to what the patient may only have been led to believe is an 'allergy' — for instance many patients complain of allergy to sticking plaster, but a test with the supposed allergenic plaster often shows that they were merely equating a sweat rash with 'allergy'.

Patients with major allergies are treated with steroids or other anti-allergic medications which will need to be continued during the perioperative period. Those with histamine mediated allergic reactions may have worse effects if given histamine releasing anaesthetic drugs. A 'history' of an allergy to any drug is an absolute contraindication to its use and probably also to drugs with similar structure. Some claims of 'allergy' e.g. gastric irritation with aspirin, are plainly not allergic in origin and can be discounted.

12. *Do you smoke?* Smoking is not welcomed by anaesthetists. No smoker can be considered healthy. Difficulties range from increased sensitivity of the airways resulting in bronchospasm, to vascular disease, premature myocardial ischaemia, and embolisation of atheromatous plaques.

Smoking must be discouraged in the 24 hours immediately preceding an anaesthetic as the resultant level of carboxyhaemoglobin will cause a significant reduction in the oxygen carrying capacity of the blood. Patients who stop smoking shortly before surgery may complain that their respiratory symptoms are worse than before, probably from recovery of the cilia, which gradually resume their function of clearing mucus from the lower respiratory tract; despite this, smokers should be encouraged to persist in abstaining to obtain the longer term benefits.

13. *Do you drink alcohol?* The excessive chronic use of alcohol is important as the resistance of the patient to other central nervous system depressants may be increased.

People are notoriously diffident about their drinking habits and the patients may not readily admit to excesses. Prolonged excess alcoholic intake causes cirrhosis, oesophageal varices, liver failure and enzyme induction, requiring increased amounts of anaesthetic drugs — all tricky anaesthetic problems.

14. *Have you ever had jaundice?* There are many causes of jaundice, but in the absence of any other proven cause (blood transfusion, biliary tract problems which result in inhibition of bile excretion, etc.) it is prudent to avoid halothane because of possible confusion with halothane hepatitis.

15. *Does arthritis or any other condition limit your neck movements or the ability to open your mouth?* If 'Yes', the anaesthetist must assess whether there will be any difficulty in intubating the patient.

16. *Do you suffer from heartburn or the return of stomach contents into your throat?* Such symptoms will alert the anaesthetist to possible increased dangers from regurgitation and pulmonary aspiration during anaesthesia.

17. *Are you pregnant?* Many drugs, including anaesthetic agents, administered during pregnancy (especially during the first trimester) may be teratogenic. The use of local anaesthetic techniques or postponement of an elective operation must be considered.

The preoperative investigations required are few for a patient with no history suggestive of electrolyte, haematological, respiratory, or myocardial upset. The following may be required depending on the extent and nature of the proposed operation.

1. *Haemoglobin.* There is some reduction of oxygen carrying capacity if the haemoglobin level is below 10 g/dl. This may

represent an increased risk in the presence of myocardial ischaemia, and will reduce the ability of the patient to withstand blood loss. It may be that a level of 8 g/dl is acceptable at the start of an operation if blood replacement is meticulous. Ideally, transfusion or supplemental iron should be given until the level of 10 g/dl is reached; 24 hours should then elapse from transfusion to allow equilibration of the cardiovascular system. The reason for the anaemia should be pursued and corrected.

2. *A sickle cell test* should be performed on patients with pigmented skin. If this is positive, special precautions are described in Chapter 12.

3. *Electrolytes*. Results of estimation of serum urea, sodium, potassium, chloride and bicarbonate should be in the normal range. A few apparently fit patients have unexpected electrolyte abnormalities which do not interfere with their normal life, but may become significant under general anaesthesia for major surgery[1].

4. *Liver function*. One in 700 apparently normal patients have preoperative abnormalities in liver function tests. This makes it worthwhile to screen all patients who are to undergo major or prolonged anaesthesia and surgery.

5. *Electrocardiogram*. All male patients over 45 years and females over 55 years should be regarded as being at risk from myocardial ischaemia. An ordinary, unstressed, electrocardiographic (ECG) investigation is unlikely to reveal abnormalities in asymptomatic patients, but it provides a reference point for comparison if ECG abnormalities arise later.

---

[1] One of the authors was faced with an apparently healthy American patient for herniorraphy, whose routine serum potassium level was reported as 7.0 (and 7.1 mmol/litre when repeated). The patient jogged, ran marathons and gave no hint of ill health. Close questioning revealed this to be chronic banana poisoning — it was his habit to eat them continuously as he exercised.

6. *Chest radiography.* The value of routine preoperative chest X-rays for fit individuals before anaesthesia is hotly debated. Surveys indicate that few abnormalities are found in patients under 30 years of age. A chest X-ray is essential before attempting endobronchial intubation, to inspect the division of the trachea into the main bronchi and to make accurate placement easier. It is worth emphasising that fit patients normally have little opportunity of a chest X-ray as a screening procedure to detect neoplasm or other abnormalities; it is therefore not unreasonable to take the opportunity when time and resources permit to make such a close examination of the chest.[2].

7. *Urine* The testing of urine in the ward is a simple, accurate and rapid procedure and usefully screens patients for glycosuria or proteinuria — each requires further investigation.

8. *Oral temperature* should be within the normal range. If it is above normal there may be a lurking infective or neoplastic disorder requiring further investigation.

9. *Weight.* All children should be weighed and this is also useful for adults as drugs are often given on a body weight basis.

Preparation for anaesthesia

The routine preparation of the fit patient for anaesthesia is fairly simple.

Starvation. Because of the danger from vomiting or regurgitation, as well as the general upset to the patient, it is normal to deny the patient all oral solids for four and preferably six hours before operation. Small quantities of clear,

---

[2] A distinguished Professor of Urology teaches that 'the examination of the chest begins and ends with a chest X-ray'. He may be right. Skilled interpretation of the X-ray is unlikely to miss any lesion of structural or functional importance.

isotonic fluids may be given to infants up to three hours pre-operatively, and up to 100 ml of water to assist the adult patient in swallowing oral premedicant drugs up to two hours before anaesthesia.

The bladder should be emptied.

Dentures and other dental furniture should be removed and the existence of other fixed prostheses such as bridges and crowns noted.

Medication may be given in advance of anaesthesia for the following purposes:

1. *Anxiolysis.* The primary purpose of premedication in contemporary practice is to allay the anxiety of the patient in the preoperative period. Medication may include hypnotics to ensure adequate sleep the night before oper-ation and a tranquil preanaesthetic period.

2. *Analgesia.* If a patient is in pain in the preoperative period the premedication should include analgesics. Many anal-gesics (including opioids) also modify mood and may be administered primarily for that purpose.

3. *Basal sedation.* In former days, when inhalation induction was routine, sedative premedication was an important factor in ensuring smooth acceptance of the anaesthetic by the patient. Since the almost routine induction of anaes-thesia by intravenous drugs, heavy preoperative sedation has become unnecessary for most adults and only rarely needed in some techniques of paediatric anaesthesia.

4. *Antisialogogue.* The reduction of the secretions of the upper respiratory tract was of utmost importance when the salivary stimulant ether was commonly employed. The need for this in premedication is less with the newer inhalational anaesthetic agents, especially if the patient is to be intubated.

5. *Vagolysis.* Vagolytic drugs, such as atropine or hyoscine, besides being antisialogogues reduce anticipated pharma-

cological or reflex effects on the heart. For example, the inhalation agent trichloroethylene or the muscle relaxant, succinylcholine, can each produce bradycardia which can be mitigated by antivagal agents. The incidence and severity of reflex cardiac irregularities produced by tracheal intubation may also be reduced after vagolytic drugs.

6. *Antiemesis.* The effect of premedication may extend to the early postoperative period after short operations. The antivagal and antisialogogue drugs hyoscine and atropine also have antiemetic actions. Antiemetics may also be required to counteract the emetic properties of opioids and other drugs in the premedicant mixture. After more drastic operations nausea is better controlled by postoperative intravenous or intramuscular injection.

7. *Antihistamines,* particularly the phenothiazines and other H_1 receptor blockers may be used to relieve or prevent the bronchospasm in patients who suffer from allergic bronchoconstriction. The phenothiazines are also often sedative, antiemetic and reduce secretions.

8. *Neutralisation of gastric acid.* The inhalation of regurgitated gastric acid and consequent pneumonitis is a dangerous complication of anaesthesia. In susceptible patients (for example pregnant women and patients with hiatus hernia) antacids or H_2 receptor blockers should be administered.

Drugs used in premedication

Premedication by intramuscular injection (between one and two hours before the induction of anaesthesia) remains the most frequent route. It must be emphasised that, apart from anxiolysis and analgesia, all the objectives of premedication listed in the last section can be achieved satisfactorily, and sometimes more reliably, by intravenous injection immediately before the induction of anaesthesia. Oral anxiolytic premedication for elective operations which do not involve the gastrointestinal tract is becoming increasingly popular.

Papaveretum and hyoscine is a mixture better known by the unofficial names of its component ('Omnopon® and Scopolamine®' or 'Om. and Scop.'). It is usually dispensed in a single ampoule and is currently the commonest intramuscular premedication administered to adults in the United Kingdom. The two drugs provide between them euphoria, anxiolysis, sedation, analgesia, cough suppression, drying of secretions, amnesia and an antiemetic effect. It is unsuitable for infants below one year of age for fear of respiratory depression, and for adults over 65 years because hyoscine may cause dysphoria as well as amnesia and undue sedation. The dose is approximately papaveretum 0.3 mg/kg and hyoscine 0.006 mg/kg but the wise anaesthetist who wishes to remain popular with the nursing staff usually prescribes it in doses which approximate to the nearest 0.25 ml of the 1 ml ampoule, (i.e. 20 mg papaveretum and 0.4 mg hyoscine (1 ml) for 60 kg adult, 15 mg and 0.3 mg (0.75 ml) for 50 kg patient, 10 mg and 0.2 mg (0.5 ml) for the 25 to 30 kg child, etc.).

Morphine and atropine is a common intramuscular premedication for older adults. It is less sedative and respiratory depressant than papaveretum, and scopolamine. Dysphoria due to the latter drug is avoided. The usual morphine dose is 10 mg scaled down to nothing between 80 and 90 years of age. The atropine component is a standard 0.6 mg for adult patients.

Pethidine, atropine and phenergan combinations have less amnesic and sedative effects than papaveretum and hyoscine unless a large dose of the phenergan component is used. Phenergan is both an antihistamine and a bronchodilator and it is thus appropriate for patients with respiratory problems or allergy. The dose of pethidine is between 1.0 to 1.5 mg/kg

(50 to 100 mg), of atropine a standard 0.6 mg and of phenergan 12.5–50 mg for the adult patient. This is a useful premedication for patients with gall bladder disease. Morphia and papaveretum both contract the biliary ducts.

Benzodiazepines. Many drugs in this category are now available. There is no advantage to giving them by injection in the healthy prepared patient; they are painful to inject and work as well if not better and more rapidly by mouth, provided the patient is sitting up and a small quantity of water is given with them. Diazepam (adult dosage 5–20 mg) is losing favour because of its long action and because its effect is prolonged by cimetidine. Lorazepam (adult dosage 2–4 mg) is shorter acting and usefully amnesic. Temazepam (adult dosage 10–30 mg) is relatively rapid in onset and short in action and thus useful for nervous outpatients.

Antihistamines for children. Oral elixirs of promethazine or trimeprazine are useful as sedatives for young children. The sugar content makes it less likely that hypoglycaemia will occur, but attracts fluid into the gastro-intestinal tract and may enhance the risk of aspiration and soiling of the lungs. The preparation Vallergan forte® contains 6 mg/ml. The dosage required is 3–4 mg/kg body weight.

Atropine (6 μg/kg) given orally is a useful drying agent before mask anaesthesia and may reduce the possibility of vagally induced dysrhythmias or bronchospasm.

H_2 *receptor blockers.* Cimetidine (200 mg), or ranitidine (150 mg) by mouth are used to prevent secretion of gastric acid and so reduce the volume and acidity of the stomach contents. The risk of acid aspiration pneumonitis is therefore reduced. Cimetidine is shorter acting but it is metabolised by the same enzyme systems as propranolol, lignocaine, and diazepam and therefore, if these drugs are also given, prolongation and potentiation of any of them may occur. Ranitidine has none of these disadvantages and lasts sufficiently long to be effective if given late on the evening before morning surgery.

Antiemetics. Emesis is one of the principal reasons for out-patients who have had non-painful minor surgery to require hospital admission. The use of preoperative oral prophylactic antiemetics like metoclopramide (adult dose 10 mg) is appro-priate in such cases.

Vasodilators. The fashion is growing of using nitroglycerine paste applied to the skin of the chest wall as prophylaxis against myocardial ischaemia. Its efficacy is not yet proven but it is an interesting concept to measure medication by the inch.[3]

The Anaesthetic

Routine checks before anaesthesia include making certain:
1. the patient's identity and the site and nature of operation.
2. that there is signed consent.
3. that there is no removable jewellery or prosthesis (including dentures).
4. that the surgeon knows the lesion, recognises the patient and is available.
5. that suction apparatus is available.
6. that drugs and apparatus for anaesthesia and resuscitation apparatus are available.
7. that trained assistance is available.
8. that hazardous infectious diseases have been excluded (e.g. Hepatitis B, HIV).

Assess and record:
1. the preoperative state.
2. the effect of premedication.

---

[3] Warnings have been issued about the possibility of explosion if defibrillator paddles are used on the chest in close proximity to the TNT paste.

3. the heart rate.
4. the systemic blood pressures
   Arrange to monitor:
1. electrocardiogram.
2. heart rate, by a peripheral pulse.
3. blood pressure by sphygmomanometer or by indwelling cannula if appropriate.
4. temperature (particularly in children) if appropriate
5. central venous pressure as appropriate.
6. oxygenation by pulse oximetry and expired carbon dioxide if apparatus is available.

The choice of anaesthetic technique must satisfy the needs of both the patient and the surgeon.

The patient expects freedom from pain (analgesia) loss of awareness and no unpleasant recall (unless he expects to be conscious under local anaesthesia).

The surgeon requires that the patient does not move nor consciously or reflexly interfere or intrude into the surgical processes of the operation, and also the provision of relaxation appropriate for the surgical procedure.

The anaesthetist must therefore ensure that the patient is unconscious (if this is appropriate) and provide analgesia by systemic or regional use of analgesic drugs, and muscle relaxation to facilitate the surgery. If neuromuscular blockers are to be used, he must be able to ventilate one or both lungs artificially.

The choice of anaesthetic, therefore, depends upon the nature and site of the operation, the patient's physical condition and the preferences and experience of the surgeon and the anaesthetist, and it must strike a balance between reduction of consciousness, abolition of pain and reduced muscle activity.

The initial choice is between general and local anaesthesia or a combination of both.

If the choice is general anaesthesia, the next decision to be made is between anaesthesia delivered from a mask or through a tube. If a tube is used ventilation can be controlled or spontaneous, but with a mask respiration should be spontaneous.

The induction of general anaesthesia by intravenous agents is nowadays usually the method of choice except for children or others with difficult veins. It is rapid and pleasant for the patient, the excitement stage and atmospheric pollution which are almost inevitable with inhalational induction are avoided, and the effects of the intravenous agents last long enough for inhalation anaesthesia to take over for easily controllable anaesthesia. But it is relatively easy to overdose the patient and cause temporary or even lethal respiratory and cardiac complications. An intravenous cannula should always be introduced and an intravenous infusion started for all but the shortest operations.

The following drugs are available for intravenous induction:

1. *Thiopentone* (4–5 mg/kg). This is the most commonly used induction agent. There is no pain on injection but it is liable to cause local venous thrombosis in some cases. The onset of anaesthesia is rapid (20 s) and smooth. I⁻ is redistributed first to the lean, and then to the fatty tissues, and then slowly released over many hours and destroyed by the liver. There is an appreciable subanaesthetic blood level which is useful while inhalational maintenance anaesthesia is established. It is liable to cause pain, thrombosis and gangrene if injected into an artery.

2. *Methohexitone* (1.0–1.3 mg/kg). There is some pain on injection and muscular twitchings and hiccoughs occur. The onset of anaesthesia is rather slower than with thiopentone but it is less irritant to veins and arteries. It also is redistributed, but the concentrations in the blood have

less subanaesthetic effect than thiopentone and it is thus useful for outpatients.

3. *Etomidate* (0.3–0.4 mg/kg). The onset of anaesthesia is rapid but there may be pain at the injection site. Muscle movement is common at induction. It is the least likely of commonly used agents to upset the cardiovascular state or release histamine. It may depress cortisol production, especially if given by infusion.

4. *Ketamine* (1–2 mg/kg). Painless and not irritant. The onset of anaesthesia is noticeably slower than thiopentone and muscular twitching and rigidity occur initially. It is a cardiovascular stimulant (blood pressures are well maintained in poor risk patients) and a bronchodilator. The margin of safety is greater, although its action lasts longer, than thiopentone (10–15 compared with 6–8 min). It is destroyed in the body and recovery to normality is rapid. If anaesthesia is maintained by inhalation for more than about 40 min after a single induction dose of ketamine, the psychic emergence reactions associated with this drug do not occur — for shorter operations they can be minimised by using a tranquilizing dose of a benzodiazepine.

5. *Propofol* (2.0–3.0 mg/kg). Onset within 30 s. Duration 4–5 min. Some pain on injection but not irritant to veins. Destroyed in the body. There is initial hypertension but it is now the drug of choice for outpatients.

6. *Benzodiazepines* may also be used, especially with poor risk patients, but the onset is slower and the dose larger compared with that needed for sedation (diazepam 0.25–0.5 mg: midazolam 0.07–0.1 mg/kg).

Inhalational induction has the advantage that the potentially frightening use of the needle can be avoided in conscious patients. The technique is particularly valuable for children and in patients with difficult veins. Oxygenation can be assured and respiration maintained throughout induction, but it is slow, an excitement phase is likely, and it is unsuitable for many adults.

Tracheal intubation or mask anaesthesia? Anaesthesia given through a tracheal tube has a number of advantages. It secures a clear airway, it facilitates artificial positive pressure ventilation for the prolonged periods required for modern muscle relaxant techniques. it permits the clearance of secretions from the trachea by suction, it provides easy surgical access to head and neck, and the scavenging of expired anaesthetic mixtures is easier than when the mask is used.

The disadvantages are that there may be anatomical difficulties which make intubation impossible, trauma to the lips, teeth, or larynx may result and, more frequently, even with the greatest care, a considerable proportion of patients will have a sore throat after intubation. Muscle relaxants (neuromuscular blocking agents) are usually used to facilitate intubation — and these, and their reversing agents, bring their own complications (see below). The physiological mechanisms of the humidification of inspired gases by the mouth and nose are also bypassed. Care must be taken to assume that the tracheal tube is not positioned unilaterally in one or other main bronchus (usually the right because of the more obtuse angle it makes with the trachea). If this is not detected, hypoxia will result because of the reduced pulmonary area for gaseous exchange whilst the cardiac output is delivered to both lungs.

Mask anaesthesia avoids the need for tracheal intubation and avoids its complications, but it is less easy to maintain a clear airway using a mask than in the intubated patient. Novices often allow air to be drawn in between the mask and the face, thus unexpectedly lightening the anaesthesia. Also, the lower respiratory tract is not isolated from the oesophagus as when the patient is intubated, and so aspiration of regurgitated gastric contents may occur.

Spontaneous respiration or controlled ventilation? Spontaneous respiration has the advantage that neither prolonged manual effort on the part of the anaesthetist nor a mechanical ventilator is required. Respiration is preserved as a useful sign of the depth of anaesthesia, and the hazard of apnoea avoided, if disconnexion of the apparatus occurs.

The disadvantages are that carbon dioxide (CO_2) retention is more likely; that the muscular work of breathing is greater than with controlled ventilation; and intrathoracic surgery is contraindicated.

Artificially controlled ventilation (intermittent positive pressure ventilation — IPPV) usually ensures adequate CO_2 elimination and adequate oxygenation. Open thorax surgery is permitted and, as neuromuscular blocking muscle relaxants are usually used to facilitate IPPV techniques, deep anaesthesia to produce muscular relaxation is unnecessary. If a degree of hypocarbia (lowered arterial carbon dioxide tension) is maintained by hyperventilation, the intracranial pressure is lowered.

The disadvantages of IPPV techniques are that the use of muscle relaxants and neostigmine and similar drugs to achieve them are not without complications and side effects, and intrathoracic pressure is raised, tending to dam back venous return and reduce cardiac output as well as introducing the occasional risk of a pneumothorax.

The use of muscle relaxants. Muscle relaxants are used to facilitate tracheal intubation by relaxing the jaw and laryngo-pharyngeal muscles and for continued muscle relaxation during surgery. The choice of drug depends on the duration of action required and a consideration of the cardiovascular effects of each agent in relation to the physical condition of the patient.

Relaxation of short duration (3–10 min) is usually obtained by the use of suxamethonium, the only depolarising agent at present in common use. The rapid onset of its action, the profound relaxation which it provides and the rapidity with which it is normally destroyed by plasma cholinesterase, make its use advantageous for intubation, whether the patient is subsequently going to breathe spontaneously during the anaesthetic or not; and rapid respiratory recovery activity is an advantage if the anaesthetist fails to intubate the patient. Suxamethonium has disadvantages: it is a depolariser (as is manifest by the fibrillation of the muscles as it takes effect) and may result in muscular pain postoperatively, especially if the patient is rapidly mobilised; it may also cause brady-cardia, especially after repeated doses; intragastric and intra-ocular pressure may be raised; it occasionally causes prolonged respiratory paralysis in individuals with impaired or deficient plasma pseudocholinesterase activity of a heredi-tary nature; there is no effective antidote and respiration must be controlled by IPPV until spontaneous reversal occurs.

Relaxation of intermediate duration (less than 25 min) can be obtained by the use of two relatively recently introduced muscle relaxants (atracurium and vecuronium) or by gall-amine, the earliest synthetic muscle relaxant. Atracurium (0.4–0.6 mg/kg) is rapidly redistributed and then destroyed by two physiological processes, Hofmann degradation and ester hydrolysis. It is therefore, useful in patients with impaired renal and hepatic function. Vecuronium (0.1–0.15 mg/kg) is rapidly redistributed and easily reversed. The amount of histamine released by either atracurium or vecuronium is small and both have minimal cardiovascular effects, although bradycardia produced by other drugs may be revealed while they are being used. Gallamine (1.5–2 mg/kg) has a similar duration. It has a vagolytic action resulting in tachycardia and a rise in blood pressure; histamine release is minimal but it is only eliminated by kidney excretion and should be avoided in gross renal disease.

Relaxation of long duration (more than 40 min) can be obtained by the use of tubocurarine, pancuronium or alcuronium. Tubocurarine (0.3–0.6 mg/kg) the original clinical muscle relaxant[4] also gives rise to autonomic ganglion blockade which often results in a fall of blood pressure.

Pancuronium (0.1 mg/kg). Increases heart rate, blood pressure and cardiac output. Alcuronium (0.2–0.3 mg/kg) has little effect on cardiovascular state.

Maintenance with inhalational agents. Anaesthetic gases and vapours are employed for maintenance of anaesthesia in the majority of general anaesthetics at the present time because of the fine control and flexibility that can be obtained by their use. Emphasis in the development of the newer agents has been on rapidity of action, speed of recovery and minimal metabolic effects. These newer agents (enflurane and isoflurane) are expensive but their advantages probably outweigh their cost.

Nitrous oxide, the first gaseous inhalation agent to be introduced, is still used today as a carrier gas in a mixture with oxygen and in concentrations up to 70%. In this concentration it usually requires supplementation with other inhalation or intravenous agents if surgical anaesthesia is to be maintained. It is, however, a useful analgesic. It is a safe agent but its main disadvantage is its lack of potency. Teratogenicity, depressive actions on the bone marrow and a destructive action on the central nervous system have been

---

[4] The history of the introduction of "Curare" into clinical practice is fascinating. The effects of the crude poison were observed by Sir Walter Raleigh when he saw it used as an arrow poison in South America in about 1596. The crude substance was brought to Europe by the flamboyant naturalist Charles Waterton, a Yorkshire squire, in 1825. He paralysed a donkey with it and rescuscitated the animal with IPPV. Claude Bernard, the great French naturalist elucidated its pharmacology in 1850. The drug was used occasionally to relieve the spasms of tetanus and in an isolated use by intramuscular injection by Lawen in 1912 for surgical relaxation. Griffith and Johnson of Montreal first used it intravenously in anaesthesia in 1942 in spontaneously breathing patients. Gray and Halton in Liverpool introduced the modern technique of paralysis and IPPV in 1946.

described after prolonged use in animals and suggested in man, but these effects have little significance within the normal time limits of anaesthesia for surgery.

Ether, the first volatile agent, to be introduced, is rarely used nowadays in anaesthetically developed environments because of its flammability, pungent smell, and cumulative effects leading to prolonged postoperative drowsiness if its concentration is not progressively reduced. It is, however, arguably the safest agent and many millions of patients owe their lives to the use of this inexpensive and universally available drug in anaesthetically deprived countries. Few cardiac irregularities result from its use, blood pressure and cardiac output are maintained and it is a bronchodilator. Its potency is low (concentrations of up to 20% are required initially) and it is irritant, which makes it a safe, but unpleasant, agent for inhalation induction.

Halothane produced a revolution in anaesthesia when it was introduced in 1956. It is potent (0.5 to 2%) and it is non-flammable, recovery is rapid and it is a bronchodilator. Its disadvantages are that it produces both respiratory and cardiac depression and there is a reduction in cardiac output and blood pressure, which can be useful to reduce surgical haemorrhage if skilfully employed. Approximately 20% of inhaled halothane is metabolised, which may be associated with very rare, but sometimes fatal, hepatic damage. Halothane can precipitate cardiac arrhythmias, especially in the presence of endogenous or exogenous adrenaline. It is a poor analgesic and will relax the pregnant uterus.

Enflurane is a non-flammable agent which is less potent than halothane (1–5%) but only 2% is metabolised and recovery is rapid and hepatitis is extremely unlikely. Cardiac arrhythmias are also rare under enflurane. Enflurane has few disadvantages, like halothane it is a respiratory depressant, but it is a better analgesic. It has caused epileptic convulsions and there is a theoretical possibility that it could cause renal damage because of its metabolism to free fluoride.

Isoflurane (0.75–2% inspired concentration) is now the most commonly used agent in the United States. It is neither flammable nor epileptogenic. It is as potent as halothane but slightly more irritant to inhale than halothane or enflurane. Like halothane and enflurane it is a respiratory depressant. It has less cardiac depressant effect and does not precipitate dysrhythmias but produces hypotension by vasodilation. It is only 0.2% metabolised and consequently has no significant hepatic or renal toxicity.

Trichloroethylene (0.35–0.5% inspired concentration) is a powerful non-flammable analgesic, but a poor anaesthetic if it is not employed with supplemental nitrous oxide. It does not depress the heart but can precipitate bradycardia and other dysrhythmias which British anaesthetists may regard as benign but Americans may consider dangerous. It does not relax the pregnant uterus, which is an advantage for certain obstetric procedures such as the removal of retained products of conception, where uterine relaxation may result in undue haemorrhage. Trichloroethylene is cumulative, it reacts with soda lime to form poisonous phosgene. Trichloroethylene has now been removed from the United States Pharmacopoea and its use in the United Kingdom is declining.

Cyclopropane (5–50% inspired concentration) is a gaseous agent which is now rarely used except by a few enthusiasts who believe that it is the best agent for the rapid inhalational induction of small children. Its main disadvantage is that it is much more explosive than ether and consequently requires elaborate safety precautions.

Chloroform (0.5–3% inspired concentration) should be mentioned for historical reasons. It virtually eclipsed ether within a year of ether being introduced in 1846 because it was potent and non-irritant when delivered by the open ('rag and bottle') method or draw over inhaler, but it has now been largely abandoned because of hepatic and cardiac toxicity.

The use of intravenous analgesics. These may be used during the maintenance of anaesthesia in patients who are artifically ventilated. After paralysis with muscle relaxants, the analgesics and nitrous oxide are given with the object of suppressing autonomic reflexes and so provide 'stress free' anaesthesia. Small doses are also used in combination with inhalational agents in spontaneously breathing patients to reduce the reflex reaction to surgical stimuli or to assist in preventing awareness.

Morphia (0.1–0.2 mg/kg), papaveretum (Omnopon) (0.1–0.3 mg/kg), pethidine (meperidine) (1.0–1.3 mg/kg), Fentanyl (1.0–3.0 μg/kg) and alfentanil (10–30 μg/kg) are used, the dosage varying according to the purpose for which the particular drug is administered. Morphine and papaveretum are relatively long acting (2–3 h) and provide excellent cardiac stability. Pethidine is shorter acting (1–2 h) and relaxes smooth muscle but it may give rise to hypotension. Fentanyl is short acting (20–40 min) and is renowned for the stability of the cardiovascular system after large doses. All are respiratory depressants — fentanyl particularly so in doses of 1.5 μg/kg or more. Alfentanil is very rapid in onset and extremely short in duration; it is therefore used primarily for brief procedures or by infusion.

Other analgesics as sufentanil, pentazocine, phenoperidine, butorphanol, meptazinol, buprenorphine, and nalbuphine are only used uncommonly in the United Kingdom as part of routine anaesthetic techniques.

Emergence from anaesthesia. Towards the end of the operation, when the surgeon begins to insert skin stitches, thought must be given to the withdrawal of the anaesthetic by, for example, gradual reduction of the inspired concentration of the inhalation agent and, when necessary, the use of specific antagonists to reverse certain categories of drugs which have been used. These antagonists include those for the reversal of competitive neuromuscular blocking muscle relaxants, and sometimes drugs which specifically oppose the central respiratory depression caused by analgesics or benzodiazepines.

The reversal of competitive muscle relaxants is essential at the end of the anaesthetic to restore the action of the muscles of respiration (the diaphragm and the intercostal muscles) in order to ensure that respiration is adequate before the patient is sent to the recovery room. The muscles of respiration are fortunately the least sensitive to the action of competitive blockers and thus the first to recover. Sometimes, particularly with the new agents atracurium and vecuronium, recovery of respiratory effort may be adequate without reversal. This is a particularly desirable cbjective if there is a bowel anastomosis, as the neostigmine, the drug used to reverse the muscle relaxant, may also cause contraction of the bowel and disruption of the anastomosis. Neostigmine (0.035–0.07 mg/kg) is usually required however, but since this drug has dangerous autonomic side effects, (bradycardia and excess bronchial and salivary secretion) a dose of atropine (0.01–0.02 mg/kg) or glycopyrrola (5–10 μg/kg) must accompany its use. It is important that there is some action in the voluntary muscles before neostigmine is administered. An electric stimulator applied to the ulnar nerve at the wrist will indicate that there is a twitch in the thumb and can be used to demonstrate full recovery of neuromuscular conduction.

Reversal of narcotic analgesics is sometimes required particularly if large doses of fentanyl have been administered. Naloxone (1.5–3 μg/kg) is usually used. Care must be taken if narcotic analgesic with actions longer than naloxone have been given since respiratory depression may return.

Non-specific stimulation of the respiratory centre is sometimes required to restore the action of the respiratory centre and start the patient breathing after prolonged IPPV, even if muscle relaxants and/or narcotic analgesics have been reversed. If the CO_2 level and respiratory drive have been reduced, carbon dioxide 5% can be administered. Doxapram (1.0–1.5 mg/kg) or the older drug, nikethamide (10–20 mg/kg) may alternatively be used for this purpose.

Extubation. If the patient has been intubated the tracheal tube has to be removed. This can be hazardous, as it converts an assured airway to one which is potentially obstructed. The patient should be turned onto his left side, the cuff around the tracheal tube is then deflated, a sucker is used to clear the pharynx around the tube under direct vision and the tube is then removed, either with manual pressure on the bag or with a catheter inserted into its lumen beyond its tip to remove secretions which have lodged between the cuff and the pharynx. The catheter technique should not be used for neurosurgical or ophthalmological patients because it may induce coughing. Finally an oropharyngeal airway is inserted.

Recovery

When the patient is on his side and breathing satisfactorily through an unobstructed airway, he may be taken to the recovery room and handed over to the recovery nurse. Oxygen should be administered on the journey if the recovery room is not immediately adjacent to the operating theatre.

The close supervision of the patient while he is recovering consciousness is a most important task and should not be delegated to an inexperienced nurse or assistant. Many deaths have occurred during this phase through neglect of simple precautions — the patient's airway may obstruct, he may vomit and inhale or he may bleed or throw himself about and injure himself. Finally, a most important duty of the recovery room nurse is to ensure that the patient is comfortable and that his pain is controlled by the injection of either intravenous or intramuscular narcotics or by other methods.

When the nurse and the anaesthetist are sure that the patient is fully conscious and in a satisfactory and stable condition, the patient is handed over to the ward staff with verbal and written details of any postoperative therapy which has been prescribed — such as intravenous fluids, antibiotics and analgesics.

Anaesthesia for elective surgery in the fit patient

The anaesthetist must select the anaesthetic technique which he considers to be the best for the treatment of the surgical condition. Often the simplest technique with which he is familiar, commensurate with the patient's safety and comfort, is most appropriate. Unnecessary overelaboration brings its own dangers.

Three techniques for the management of a fit 50–70 kg adult for various conditions are given as examples but, it must be emphasised, in each case they represent only one of several possible methods of management.

Anaesthesia for a day-stay diagnostic dilatation and curettage

The problem. The patient requires to be restored to near normality immediately postoperatively so that she can be sent home to recuperate after a few hours. The shortest acting agents must be used.

Assessment. The patient is known to be fit and any necessary investigations such as haemoglobin estimation should have been carried out in advance, but nevertheless the history should be checked and the patient examined. Any acute condition such as a sore throat or common cold should be diagnosed and the anaesthetic postponed.

Preparation. The patient should have been warned in advance not to have taken food or drink by mouth but this should be checked by direct questioning. The bladder should be emptied immediately before anaesthesia.

Premedication. Paradoxically, sedative premedicant drugs often act for longer than the anaesthetic. Premedication is not usually necessary, but if the patient is very nervous a small dose of a benzodiazepine may be given — for example, 10 mg temazepam, or 0.125 mg triazolam orally with a sip of water.

Many anaesthetists today feel that the stomach should be emptied pharmacologically preoperatively (by the oral administration of metoclopramide (10 mg)) and the volume and acidity of the gastric contents reduced by a dose of 150 mg of ranitidine orally two hours before anaesthesia.

Monitoring. The blood pressure should be taken in advance of surgery and the cuff left in place. An electrocardiograph is attached to monitor the heart. A pulse oximeter is advisable if available.

Induction. An indwelling needle or cannula is inserted. One of the short duration agents such as methohexitone or propofol should be used — up to about 100 mg and 200 mg, respectively, for a 60–70 kg patient. A good tip is to administer half the calculated dose rapidly, and then to titrate the remainder according to the response of the patient, as demonstrated by the abolition of the eyelash reflex.

Maintenance. The mask is applied with the pop-off valve open with a gas flow of 10 l/min (oxygen 3 l/min and nitrous oxide 7 l/min) using a Magill, Bain or Lack system (Chapter 7). A brief period of apnoea when it may be necessary to squeeze the reservoir bag gently may follow the administration of the induction agents. The volatile agent is next gradually introduced (halothane, enflurane or isoflurane at 0.25%) and its concentration is increased in 0.5% increments every 4 breaths to halothane 2%, enflurane 4% or isoflurane 2.5%.

If the eyelash reflex is absent, the eyelid may be gently opened; the pupil should be small and unresponsive and possibly divergent. An oropharyngeal airway is inserted to keep the tongue forward and the mouth open. The patient may now be placed in the lithotomy position and the surgeon can begin. The response of the patient to the surgical stimulus is observed: if the respiratory rate or depth increased markedly or the patient holds her breath or the heart rate increases, a small dose of alfentanil (0.25–0.5 mg) may be useful.

Emergence. As surgery is completed the nitrous oxide is turned off, 7 l/min of 100% oxygen is administered and the patient is turned on her left side with a 15% head-down tilt and taken to the recovery room, where oxygen administration is continued.

Recovery. When the patient responds to commands and rejects her airway, she can be turned into the supine position and be allowed to sit up, first on the trolley, then in a chair. Finally, when she is orientated in time and space and steady on her feet, she may be allowed to go home, accompanied by a responsible and instructed adult who will supervise the patient for at least 24 h, during which time she should not drive a car or operate machinery (including cookers). A supply of an oral analgesic such as paracetamol in 1000 mg doses may be required.

Anaesthesia for a small benign nodule of the thyroid gland.

The problem. The operation is a 'body surface' procedure for which the patient can breathe spontaneously but tracheal intubation will be required to allow the surgeon easy access. The patient is to remain in hospital after the operation.

Assessment and preparation as for the first example.

Premedication: Sedative premedication can be given, as the patient is to stay in hospital overnight; papaveretum 20 mg and hyoscine 0.4 mg would be satisfactory. Medication to reduce the potential hazards of regurgitation may be given as in the first example.

Monitoring should include the items mentioned in the first example.

Induction. An infusion of Hartmann's solution should be started. Induction can be with the longer acting agent thio-

pentone (300–400 mg for a 60–70 kg adult) administered in
a similar manner to that described in the first example. This
is followed by the short-acting muscle relaxant suxamethonium (75–100 mg). If a small dose of the neuromuscular
blocking drug tubocurarine is given immediately before thiopentone, the incidence of postoperative muscle pains due to
the suxamethonium will be reduced.

Apnoea rapidly follows the administration of suxamethonium after depolarising muscle fibrillation produced by the
succinycholine. An oropharyngeal airway can be inserted if
necessary to keep the airway clear, and the patient is ventilated via a mask with a 50% : 50% mixture of oxygen and
nitrous oxide from a Magill, Bain or Lack system, to ensure
oxygenation and anaesthesia during laryngoscopy and intubation. Care is taken to observe the movement of the chest
and the electrocardiograph trace. A simple added precaution
is for the attendant nurse to keep a finger on the pulse.

Laryngoscopy and intubation. The glottis and cords of the well
oxygenated patient are exposed. The cords may then be
sprayed with 4% lignocaine (up to 5 ml or 1 mg/kg) to reduce
the hypertensive response to intubation, after which the
patient is intubated and the cuff on the tube is blown up[1].
Intermittent inflation with 50% N_2O : O_2 mixture continues
while both lungs are auscultated to ensure that the tube has
not been passed too far and entered a bronchus.

Maintenance. The respiratory muscles gradually repolarise
and the patient begins to breathe. A mixture of 3 l/min of
oxygen and 7 l/min of nitrous oxide is now breathed spontaneously, to which 2% halothane, 4% enflurane or 3%
isoflurane is gradually added. If the patient holds his breath,
'bucks' or moves, an additional increment of thiopentone can

---

[1] The technique of oral tracheal intubation is described and illustrated
in Chapter 14 (Figure 14.2).

be given or fentanyl 50–100 μg may be cautiously administered, care being taken not to produce apnoea.

Emergence, extubation and recovery will be as already described earlier in this chapter. Intramuscular narcotic analgesics may be required in the initial stages followed by oral analgesics.

Anaesthesia for the excision of a small ovarian cyst.

The problem. This is a relatively minor operation for a fit patient. Blood loss will be minimal but abdominal muscular relaxation will be required throughout the surgical procedure.

Assessment, preparation and examination will be as for the two earlier examples.

Premedication may be with a opioid — and hyoscine or atropine, or an oral benzodiazepine can be used. The opioid has the advantage that, with this relatively short operation, some analgesia may persist into the immediate postoperative period. If oral benzodiazepines are chosen a preoperative injection will be avoided.

An intravenous infusion of Hartmann's Ringer lactate solution should be set up: 500 ml can be given in the first hour to replace the pre-existing fluid deficit from starvation, and after that, the rate should be approximately 100 ml/h plus approximately 2 ml for every 1 ml blood estimated to have been lost. Monitoring will be as discussed for the previous example.

Induction, laryngoscopy and intubation could be as in the last example, with suxamethonium used intially as the relaxant for intubation, but many anaesthetists would prefer to use the longer acting, competitive relaxant chosen for subsequent maintenance — for example, vecuronium 6 mg for a 60–70 kg adult. Ventilation with 50% nitrous oxide : oxygen mixture would have to be continued for a little longer (2–3 min) with the competitive agents, and conditions for intubation may not be so good as with suxamethonium; the 4% lignocaine spray should be used as previously described.

Maintenance. Fentanyl 50–100 μg can be given either with the induction dose of thiopentone or after intubation. If suxamethonium was given for intubation, vecuronium 5 mg is given as soon as the patient starts to breathe spontaneously. If vecuronium has been given for intubation the patient will remain apnoeic. In either case, the patient should be ventilated at 10 ml/kg (600–700 ml for a 60–70 kg adult) at 10–12 breaths per min, either by hand or with a mechanical ventilator. The tidal volume should be checked with a respirometer and the inflation pressure should not exceed 25 cm H_2O. The anaesthetic mixture should be 30% oxygen and 70% nitrous oxide with a low concentration of halothane (0.25–0.5%), enflurance (0.5–1.0%), or isoflurane (0.25–0.5%) to avoid recall.

Increments of 1–2 mg of vecuronium will be required after 30 min when signs of spontaneous respiration begin to recur. Additional doses of fentanyl (50–100 μg) may be necessary.

Emergence, including reversal of the neuromuscular blocking agents, and extubation will be as described earlier in the chapter.

Recovery room care must include the administration of analgesics and, if necessary, antiemetics, and careful assessment of the vital signs of blood pressure and pulse to guard against any possibility of haemorrhage.

9

Local and regional anaesthesia

'. . . chloroform has done a lot of mischief. It's enabled every
fool to be a surgeon'
Sir Patrick Cullen in *The Doctor's Dilemma*
George Bernard Shaw (1856–1950).

It is probably true that local anaesthesia is used less often
than it should be in the United Kingdom, particularly for
major surgery. This may be because physicians have always
been responsible for the administration of general anaesthesia.
The fact that local anaesthesia may be appreciably safer than
general anaesthesia in certain circumstances, or lead to fewer
unpleasant postoperative side effects in others, is often
ignored in favour of the comparative speed and ease of
administration of general anaesthesia. It is true that no one
can absolutely guarantee the success of a local anaesthetic
administered to a conscious patient, but given time, trouble
and practice, and the careful selection of the appropriate techniques, reliability can almost be guaranteed. It is sad that
many anaesthetists are not prepared to spend time and
trouble learning the art of administering local anaesthesia. It
is sadder still that some of those who will not bother to learn
are most vociferous in belittling its efficacy, and that their
prejudice is easily spread to surgeons, nurses and patients.

Local anaesthesia is, however, currently enjoying a modest
increase in popularity. The introduction of longer acting local

anaesthetic agents like bupivacaine has led to the realisation that its use, even in a 'single shot' technique can be of real benefit in providing relaxation and analgesia under general anaesthesia, and postoperative pain relief for the critical period after surgery; thus, there is good reason to practice and teach techniques of local anaesthesia under the cover of general anaesthesia. The revolution in the provision of obstetric analgesia and anaesthesia is another factor; first pudendal block effectively replaced the use of general anaesthesia for forceps delivery, and then caudal and subsequently epidural techniques became increasingly popular — initially for analgesia for delivery *per vaginam* and then for caesarean section. Few would have thought twenty years ago that a movement for the participation of both father and mother in the process of labour, and emphasis on the importance of early 'bonding' between mother and child, would have led to the growing demand by both obstetrician and patient for caesarean section under epidural anaesthesia with the father present.

Rapport and sedation

Successful local anaesthesia, with the patient conscious, requires deliberate and sympathetic rapport with the patient, meticulous attention to detail, the wholehearted cooperation of both the surgeon and the nursing staff and the judicious use of supplementary analgesics and sedatives. It should be remembered that some sedatives (the benzodiazepines for example) may have sedative and amnesic effects which last for far longer than the general anaesthesia produced by some modern short acting intravenous and inhalational agents. It is often better to use shorter acting techniques, such as the inhalation of nitrous oxide and oxygen mixtures or minimal incremental doses of pethidine or other analgesics.

Indications for local or regional anaesthesia

1. *If the life of the patient would be endangered by unconsciousness*, for example by respiratory obstruction or pulmonary infection.
2. *Emergencies when there is no time to reduce the hazards of general anaesthesia.* This would apply in certain cases of 'full stomach' and operative obstetric delivery, and in some cases of diabetes, myasthenia gravis, sickle cell disease, advanced old age, or debility, and for prolonged surgery for reimplantation of severed digits.
3. *To avoid hazards of administering general anaesthetic drugs.* For example, in acute intermittent porphyria, repeated halothane anaesthesia, myotonia, and renal or hepatic failure.
4. *Procedures requiring patient's cooperation*, as some tendon repairs, eye operations and in pharyngeal motility studies.
5. *Minor superficial and body surface lesions*, like uncomplicated dental extraction, skin lesions, minor lacerations and scar revision.
6. *To provide postoperative analgesia.* Particular examples are circumscision, thoracotomy, herniorraphy, skin graft donor sites and abdominal surgery.
7. *To produce sympathetic blockade*, as in free flap or reimplantation surgery, or limb ischaemia.
8. *If the patient or surgeon or the anaesthetist has a preference for local anaesthesia* and can convince the other parties that local anaesthesia is appropriate.

Contraindications to the use of local anaesthesia

1. *Known allergy or hypersensitivity to local anaesthetic drugs.* This is rare indeed — most so called reactions are either due to overdose or intravascular injection.
2. *Lack of skilled personnel* capable of undertaking and/or

supporting a particular technique. There are certain techniques which require only a minimum amount of knowledge or training, for example, the 'infiltration, cut and sew' techniques, or the application of topical anaesthesia. There are others which, once they have been learned and their particular dangers have been appreciated, can be relatively easily repeated with a considerable chance of success because the correct placement of the needle is indicated by a definite sign — for example by withdrawal of blood in regional intravenous anaesthesia or cerebrospinal fluid (CSF) in spinal anaesthesia. Most peripheral nerve blocks and lumbar or caudal (sacral) epidurals need training, persistence and constant practice.

Well informed assistance is desirable either for positioning the patient for the placing of the needle (epidurals and brachial plexus blocks, for example), or for managing an expected side effect like hypotension in subarachnoid spinal anaesthesia.

3. *Lack of resuscitation facilities.* It is foolhardy to believe that complications can never happen (e.g. hypersensitivity, relative overdose, pneumothorax in supraclavicular or intercostal block, failure of the arterial cuff in regional intravenous anaesthesia or dural puncture during an attempted epidural). It is accepted practice that resuscitation equipment and a full range of emergency drugs must be immediately available in modern hospitals. The extent that they are required in other situations depends on the technique chosen and the anatomical region operated upon.

Some techniques require specific procedures to combat expected side effects almost as a routine. One example is the need for the prevention or treatment of hypotension in subarachnoid spinal anaesthesia. The injection of local anaesthesia around nerves in the limbs or extremities is less likely to cause complications than injection into the trunk or head and neck.

4. *Local infection or ischaemia at the site of injection.* Local acidosis will mitigate against the effect of injected local anaesthetic agents, quite apart from the danger of the spread of infection. Nerves remote from, but supplying the infected site, can of course still safely be blocked. In some areas infection of the skin will contraindicate injection into a deeper area — infection at the site of a proposed lumbar puncture for example.

5. *Extensive surgery which will require toxic doses of local anaesthetic.* The blood levels from an abdominal field block may be safe for a fit subject but might cause a dangerous reduction in cardiac output in an elderly patient with a poor myocardium.

6. *Anatomical distortion or cicatrix formation.*

7. *The risk of haematoma in certain sites* (e.g. the epidural space) from medication with anticoagulants, a bleeding tendency or haemophilia.

8. *If immediate anaesthesia is required* (for example an obstructed breech delivery) or there is not sufficient time for the local anaesthetic to act properly.

9. *Lack of consent or cooperation on the part of the patient.* Provided the anaesthetist is demonstrably confident, most British patients will usually accept the advice to have local anaesthesia, particularly if there are good reasons for avoiding general anaesthesia. It is unwise to persuade a patient to have local anaesthesia if the only reason is to indulge the anaesthetist's need to practice that particular technique. On the other hand, under United Kingdom law, the process of obtaining informed consent does not require the anaesthetist to scare the patient stiff by reciting a litany of all the complications which may ensue however remote, whenever he is about to administer either local or

general anaesthesia. It is sufficient for him to advise that, in his professional opinion, and in his hands, the procedure he is proposing is safe and reasonable in the circumstances.

Local anaesthesia is not generally a good alternative to general anaesthesia for the mentally deranged or pathologically frightened patient, nor for a patient who does not speak the same language — an interpreter has to be exceptionally experienced to get the anaesthetist's message across to the patient. The use of local anaesthesia alone in children is unusual in British practice except for some dental procedures and minor surgery, but in sympathetic and expert hands it can be used satisfactorily without producing mental trauma.

Local anaesthetic agents

The most commonly used local anaesthetic agents in the United Kingdom are lignocaine, prilocaine and bupivacaine. All are amide linked local anaesthetics. In addition, cocaine, a natural ester alkaloid, is used for surface anaesthesia in 5% to 10% solution.

Lignocaine is used for all but the most major surgery when analgesia is required for some hours into the post operative period. It is rapid in onset and its action persists for 90 to 120 min with adrenaline and up to 90 minutes without. Lignocaine is used for infiltration and peripheral nerve blocks in 0.5%, 1%, 1.5% and 2% solution, as a 4% solution for topical anaesthesia, and as a 5% heavy solution in dextrose for subarachnoid blocks. The maximum safe dose is 7 mg/kg body weight with adrenaline and 3 mg/kg without.

Prilocaine is very similar to lignocaine except its toxicity is less and its onset is slightly slower. Its duration is also a little longer. The drug is used in similar strengths to lignocaine but its maximum safe doses are 9 mg/kg body weight with adrenaline and 6 mg/kg without. Its most important uses are when large volumes of agent are required or for deliberate intravenous injection in regional intravenous anaesthesia (see below).

Bupivacaine is slower in onset and longer in duration than lignocaine because it has a greater ability to bind to protein. Bupivacaine is ideal when a long action is required but, being protein bound, adrenaline has no effect on the amount which can be given (maximum safe dose with or without adrenaline 2 mg/kg body weight). It is, however, more potent than lignocaine (strengths 0.125% to 0.5%) and the volumes of 0.5% solution that can be given are roughly equivalent to the use of 1.5% lignocaine with adrenaline.

Adrenaline is added to local anaesthetic solutions in strengths of 1 : 80,000 to 1 : 500,000 to delay absorption of the solution at the site of action. This increases the rate of onset of action, prolongs the duration and reduces the likelihood of high blood levels which may cause toxic reactions. Adrenaline also directly counteracts the depressant effect on the heart of the local agent absorbed into the blood stream. Thus, unless the particular drug is also protein bound, as is bupivacaine, larger doses can be given in the presence of adrenaline than without it. If the infiltration technique is used, adrenaline helps the surgeon by producing local vasoconstriction.

The effect of adrenaline is not wholly benign. It may have cardiac effects (particularly if injected intravascularly and/or in the presence of halothane) which include ventricular ectopics, ventricular fibrillation, tachycardia, hypertension and myocardial ischaemia. It should never be used for ring blocks of the digits or penis as necrosis may result constriction of the end arteries. Local ischaemia from adrenaline in infected areas may predispose to anaerobic infection.

Dangers, side effects and toxicity of local anaesthetic agents

Hypersensitivity reactions to local anaesthetic agents are rare with the amide agents. Procaine, an ester based anaesthetic, had a reputation for causing dermal hypersensitivity reactions but major anaphylactic responses such as those described in Chapter 13 were unusual.

Absolute and relative overdosage giving rise to toxic responses occur more easily with local anaesthetics than with other drugs because of the manner in which they are employed. The main effects of high concentrations of local anaesthetics absorbed or injected into the blood stream are on the brain (with lignocaine — first depression and then convulsions) and on the heart — cardiovascular and myocardial depression and vasolidation. The formerly widely used ester agents, of which procaine was the most popular, are destroyed by cholinesterases in the blood, so toxic reactions were comparatively rare because high blood levels were less likely. Modern amide local anaesthetics are different, being destroyed more slowly by the liver. It soon became apparent when lignocaine was introduced in the 1950s that greater attention had to be paid to keeping within the maximum safe dosage as the incidence of toxic reactions increased.

Some techniques are known to cause high blood levels because of the vascularity of the region into which they are injected and the comparatively large dose of agent required. These include intercostal block, and lumbar and caudal epidural blocks. The beneficial effects of adding adrenaline solutions have been noted above. Intravascular injection must be avoided at all costs: it gives rise to immediate high blood levels. The important rules are always to aspirate before injecting and to keep the needle moving during infiltration techniques.

Signs and symptoms of toxic overdose. Often the first signs of an excessive blood level of local anaesthetic is numbness of the tongue and around the mouth. Ester anaesthetics (including procaine and cocaine) initially tend to make the patient anxious and excited, but with amides like lignocaine the first sign of overdosage is often drowsiness. Muscular twitchings follow; these are first noticed around the eyes. Some patients complain of a feeling of impending doom, and if the danger is ignored and the patient is left untreated, convulsions may follow. Depression of the myocardium and vasodilation occur at the same time, causing hypotension. Cardiac arrest and apnoea may follow.

Treatment. Oxygen is administered — under pressure by face mask if the patient breathes inadequately. An intravenous infusion is set up. The patient may need to be intubated and ventilated. Muscular twitchings and convulsions may be treated with continuously administered intravenous thiopentone or a benzodiazepine. Ephedrine may be required to counteract hypotension both by stimulating the myocardium and combatting peripheral vasodilation. The airway must be protected. Intubation and artificial ventilation may be necessary if the patient does not breath adequately.

Preparation and precautions before the use of local anaesthesia

1. *Formal explanation and verbal consent* with identification of the part to be operated upon.
2. *Starvation* except for the most minor procedures, especially if supplementary sedation is a possibility.
3. *Indwelling intravenous needle* — with infusion for more major surgery, or if sympathetic paralysis is likely.
4. *Heart rate, blood pressure,* and electrocardiographic monitoring.
5. *Check the oxygen supply, emergency drugs and apparatus.*

6. *Check supplementary drugs and apparatus for systemic analgesia and sedation.*

Topical anaesthesia

Surface anaesthesia for mucous and other membranes for procedures involving superficial cutting or for diagnostic instrumentation. Sites include: eyes (conjunctiva) nasal cavity, throat, larynx, lower respiratory tract, the ear (for emergency paracentesis of the ear drum), the urethra and the birth canal. Applicaton is by instillation (urethra), spray (pressure or aerosol) or ointments, pastes and gels. A recent innovation is Emla® cream — a mixture of lignocaine and prilocaine for application to the skin before venepuncture; this is especially valuable for children but takes 1 hour to act.

The agents usually used are lignocaine 4% (maximum 5 ml for a 70 kg man) and cocaine 5% (maximum 5 ml for 70 kg man). Cocaine is also vasoconstrictive.

Infiltration

Superficial injection into or around a lesion to block sensory nerve endings for body surface surgery is a simple, familiar and reliable technique.

The technique of 'infiltrate and cut' for the skin and subcutaneous layers was much used in the past in anaesthetically underdeveloped countries. The technique was not only used for limb amputations and the like but also for opening the abdomen. Almost unlimited quantities of dilute solutions of procaine could be used because it is destroyed locally by enzymes in the blood and not by the liver as is the case with amide anaesthetics.

Infiltration should also be used in the line of an incision for major surgery if the patient is conscious after nerve trunks have been blocked proximally. This is desirable so that the sensitive nerve endings immediately beneath the skin are adequately anaesthetised. The addition of adrenaline aids the surgeon by reducing bleeding.

Direct injection into a fracture haematoma is also used. It is simple and effective especially when backed by systemic intravenous or inhalational analgesia.

Intravenous regional anaesthesia (Bier's block)

This is a simple and reliable technique for producing anaesthesia of a whole limb — usually the upper. Careful attention to detail is necessary if dire complications are to be avoided. Resuscitation equipment should always be to hand as large volumes of local anaesthetic are used. The technique is applicable to patients who can safely have an arterial tourniquet applied. It is, therefore, contraindicated in patients with sickle cell disease, peripheral vascular disease or diabetes (see Chapter 12.)

An indwelling intravenous cannula is first placed in a vein of the opposite hand as a precaution against emergencies. A similar cannula is then inserted on the back of the hand of the limb which is to be operated upon. The limb is then exsanguinated either by elevation for 3 min while pressure is kept on the brachial artery, or by an elastic rubber (Esmarch) tourniquet if this is tolerated by the patient. The cuff is then inflated to 100 mmHg above the level of the patient's arterial systolic pressure. Next 30–40 ml (0.75 ml/kg) of prilocaine 0.5% *without adrenaline* is injected into the intravenous cannula.

Prilocaine is usually recommended because a large volume of local anaesthetic is to be injected intravenously and it is less toxic than lignocaine. Bupivacaine should not be used, because if it should get past the cuff, it will bind with the heart muscle, being a protein bound drug, and may cause cardiac arrest which is resistant to treatment. Local anaesthetic will pass the tourniquet if the cuff is defective and deflates, if the injection is made too vigorously into the vein and the solution is forced under the cuff and, possibly, through abnormally large nutrient arteries to the humerus. The cuff should be kept inflated for at least 20 min whatever the length of the operation, otherwise the concentration of the local anaesthetic in the blood will reach an unacceptably high level when it is deflated. Double cuffs are sometimes used, the lower cuff being inflated on the anaesthetised area and the upper cuff then being deflated — however, most patients tolerate a single cuff remarkably well for up to 45 min.

Nerve blocks for the upper limb

The brachial plexus originates in the neck from the anterior divisions of the fifth, sixth, seventh and eighth cervical and the first thoracic nerve. The three principal nerves of the upper limb (radial, medial and ulnar) are formed from the three cords around the axillary artery. The plexus is encased in a conical sheath of fascia which extends from the vertebrae to the axillary artery. The sheath thus encloses virtually the whole nerve supply of the upper limb including the shoulder. The objective of brachial plexus block, whatever approach is used, is to enter the sheath with a needle and to fill it with local anaesthetic, thus blocking the entire plexus and its branches; 30–40 ml of solution are required in the adult.

The sheath may be entered between the anterior and medical scalene muscles in the neck ('interscalene' approach) as the plexus crosses the first rib behind the clavicle ('supraclavicular approach'), or in the axilla as the cone narrows down to invest the artery ('axillary approach'). Injection into a blood vessel is avoided, as with all nerve blocks, by aspiration before injection. Careful technique will minimise the danger of entering the pleura in the neck during a supraclavicular approach. The use of a peripheral nerve stimulator to locate the plexus, and even its individual trunks, greatly improves the success of these blocks. Sometimes septa within the sheath may result in uneven distribution of the drug and patchy analgesia in the limb.

The radial, median and ulnar nerves ultimately supply the dorsum, lateral and medial areas of the palmar aspect of the hand respectively. The three nerves may be blocked individually at the elbow or at the wrist.

Digital nerve block is perhaps the block used most frequently in Accident and Emergency Departments. Even this simple block can be a very uncomfortable experience for the patient if it is not carried out properly. It is possible to block all four nerves to a digit through one needle puncture.

Nerve blocks to the lower limb and pudendal area

There is no convenient single sheath like the brachial sheath round all the nerves of the lumbar and sacral plexuses. The pudendal nerve supplies the perineum. Five separate nerves supply the skin, muscles and joints of the leg. The femoral and lateral cutaneous nerve of thigh pass anteriorly under the inguinal ligament, the obturator nerve reaches the thigh through the obturator foramen; all three are derived from the lumbar roots. The sciatic and posterior cutaneous nerve of the thigh (from the lower lumbar and sciatic roots) pass through the greater sciatic notch posteriorly. The femoral nerve supplies the front of the thigh and the medial aspect of the leg to the instep, the obturator nerve the inner aspect of the thighs. The sciatic and posterior cutaneous nerves of thigh, running together supply the posterior aspect of the leg and thigh, together with the lateral side of the leg and both the dorsum and the sole of the foot. The femoral nerve can be blocked just below the inguinal ligament, where it is lateral to the femoral artery, and the lateral cutaneous nerve of thigh just below the anterior superior iliac spine. The approach to the obturator nerve is not easy, but if sufficient local solution (30 ml) is injected into the femoral sheath it will track back to the lumbar roots and block both obturator and femoral. The sciatic nerve can be blocked either from a posterior approach or from the anterior aspect employing a somewhat complicated geometric construction which also enables the femoral nerve to be blocked in Hunter's canal *pari passu*.

The ankle block is another useful technique for the lower limb. This technique blocks four branches of the sciatic nerve which supply the foot. These are the anterior tibial anteriorly midway between the malleoli, the musculocutaneous, superficially between the malleoli, the posterior tibial behind the medial malleolus and the sural behind the lateral malleolus. The saphenous branch of the femoral must also be blocked (anterior to the medial malleolus). Digital blocks may also be used for the toes.

The pudendal nerve, supplying the outlet of the birth canal, is related to the spine of the ischium. It can be blocked *per vaginam* by palpating the spine or through the buttock with a finger locating the spine *per rectum*. The branches of the pudendal nerve supplying the penis can be blocked at the base of the organ.

Nerve blocks of the thorax and abdomen

The intercostal nerves supply the skin and muscles of the thorax and abdomen. The intercostal nerves lie in a groove on the inside of the lower border of each rib, they are best blocked in the midscapula line so that their lateral cutaneous branches can be included; care must be taken to avoid causing pneumothorax, and aspiration is crucial to eliminate the risk of intravascular injection into the intercostal blood vessels which are closely associated with the nerves.

Intercostal thoracic nerves 6 to 10 supply the skin and muscles of the upper abdomen from the xiphisternum to the umbilicus, and thoracic 10 to 12 the skin and muscles of the lower abdomen. Upper abdominal laparotomy can be undertaken under local anaesthesia if intercostal block is combined with a block of the vagus nerve at the cardia of the stomach and of the coeliac plexus between the aorta and the vena cava as soon as the abdomen is opened.

The ilioinguinal and iliohypogastric nerves (thoracic 12 and lumbar 1 roots) supply the inguinal region. They can be blocked by piercing the exterior oblique aponeurosis just inside the anterior superior iliac spine. This block plus infiltration over the inguinal ligament and direct vision injection of the neck of the sac is the basis of local block for hernia operations. This is a most useful technique, particularly for elderly patients with cardiopulmonary problems.

Nerve blocks of the head and neck

The terminal branches of the divisions of the trigeminal nerve can be blocked as they emerge from foramina (such as the infra- and supraorbital externally and the inferior dental inside the mouth for dental procedures).

The trunks of the three divisions of the trigeminal nerve can be blocked at the base of the skull by those who are practised. The pterygopalatine block is perhaps the most useful of these techniques; it not only blocks the upper jaw and teeth but also the inside of the maxilla including the sinuses.

Blocks for eye surgery are a specialist subject but they include retrobulbar block, which anaesthetises the extraocular muscles, and block of the facial nerve just in front of the tragus of the ear, which relaxes the muscles of the eyelids and avoids blepharospasm.

The anatomy of the vertebral column and spinal cord and its investing membrane

The spinal cord begins at the foramen magnum as a continuation of the medulla oblongata and extends to the level of the first or second lumbar vertebra. It is closely invested by a membrane called the pia mater and is surrounded by cerebrospinal fluid (CSF) which is in direct continuity with the CSF surrounding the brain. The CSF is contained in a space enclosed by a double membrane — an outer fibrous membrane (the dura mater) with a thin transparent membrane (the arachnoid mater) closely applied to its inner surface. The space between these, (the 'subdural' space) is normally only a potential space and of limited practical importance. The space containing the CSF between the arachnoid and the spinal cord invested by the pia mater is known either as the 'subarachnoid space' or the 'intradural space'. The dura (and thus the subarachnoid space) extends as a tube ending blindly at the level of the second sacral vertebra.

The spinal nerve roots to the segments of the body below the foramen magnum leave the cord and pass across the subarachnoid space. There are 8 cervical nerves, 12 thoracic, 5 lumbar, 5 sacral and 1 coccygeal nerve. Because the spinal cord ends at the level of L2 in the adult all nerve roots below the second lumbar (i.e. those which form the lumbar and sacral plexuses and supply the legs and perineum) pass almost vertically downwards to the subarachnoid in a bundle, appropriately known as the 'cauda equina' (horse's tail) before leaving their respective intervertebral foramina. In this region the nerves are bathed in CSF, and it is here that the subarachnoid space is most easily entered by a needle inserted between the lumbar vertebrae, and local anaesthetic is injected to produce a spinal (subarachnoid) block. All the thoracic nerves (T1 to T12) carry sympathetic vasoconstrictor fibres.

The epidural (or extradural) space lies within the bony vertebral canal between the dura, and the periosteum lining the inside of the lamina of the vertebra. The periosteum and the dura are fused at the foramen magnum thus closing the space superiorly. By contrast the subarachnoid space is in continuity with the cranial cavity. The epidural space is limited inferiorly by the sacral hiatus closed by the sacrococcygeal membrane at the apex of the sacral bone. The epidural space contains the spinal nerves as they pass to their respective foramina, and also contains alveolar tissue, arteries and a plexus of veins.

The part of the epidural space contained within the bony sacral canal is known as the caudal (or sacral) epidural space. As the dura containing the CSF ends at S2 in the adult, there is a space between it and the sacrococcygeal membrane into which local anaesthetic injections can be made with comparative safety through the sacrococcygeal membrane.

The paravertebral spaces in the thoracic region are bounded above and below by the periosteum of the ribs and laterally by the costotransverse ligaments. Each thoracic paravertebral space transmits the respective intercostal nerve from the intervertebral foramen on its way to the intercostal space. Individual paravertebral spaces do not communicate directly with the spaces above and below, but indirectly through the epidural space via the intervertebral foramina. In the lumbar region, communication between spaces is more open.

Nomenclature of spinal and extradural blocks

It will be obvious from the number of alternate words given above that there is a considerable variability in the forms by which the various spaces and injections are known. There does, however, seem to be wide agreement about the term 'paravertebral'. The most logical system for the other spaces and blocks is probably 'spinal intradural' for injections into the CSF 'spinal extradural' for injections into the extradural (epidural) space via the space between the vertebrae and 'sacral' or 'caudal extradural' for injections via the sacrococcygeal membrane. The forms 'spinal', 'epidural' and 'caudal' are, however, deeply rooted in the colloquial anaesthetic vocabulary. In this chapter the compromise of using the descriptions 'spinal subarachnoid', 'lumbar (or thoracic) epidural', and 'caudal' blocks will be adopted.

Spinal subarachnoid block

This is one of the earliest and most reliable and effective techniques.

Advantages
1. There is definite evidence that the needle tip has been placed in the correct position (by withdrawal of cerebrospinal fluid).
2. Only a small volume of local anaesthetic is needed because of the fluid nature of CSF — this virtually eliminates the possibility of toxicity from overdose.

Disadvantages and contraindications.
1. The danger of infection causing meningitis when the needle has been inserted through carefully prepared skin has been almost eliminated by modern methods of sterilisation (autoclaving, ethylene oxide, and irradiation) and the provision of disposable sterile packs. Injection into the CSF through an infected area is absolutely contraindicated.
2. The incidence of 'spinal headache' attributed to leakage of CSF after the withdrawal of the needle has been reduced, but not eliminated, by the use of fine spinal needles (25 and 26g).
3. The block usually involves sympathetic paralysis in the upper lumbar and lower thoracic regions. Hypotension is the result of vasodilation unless counter measures are used ('preloading' with intravenous colloids or crystalloids and

the use of vasopressors like ephedrine). Saddle block (see below) is low enough to avoid this complication.

4. The injection of too large a volume of local anaesthetic or an unexpectedly high spread can cause prolonged respiratory paralysis. This complication necessitates artificial ventilation.

5. Damage to the cord or to spinal nerve roots, whether from direct trauma or spasm of the arteries supplying the cord, or from hypotension, is rare except if some solution other than a local anaesthetic is injected. Spinal anaesthesia should not be used in the presence of active neurological spinal disease. The evidence whether or not spinal subarachnoid block really exacerbates such conditions is equivocal; but it is best avoided as any worsening of the condition will otherwise assuredly be blamed on the procedure.

6. Urinary retention is possible after spinal anaesthesia. If the patient had a degree of outflow obstruction before surgery, temporary insertion of a catheter may be all that is required; but in males resection of the prostate may be necessary.

7. Backache occurs frequently after spinal anaesthesia, especially if repeated attempts at lumbar puncture have been necessary.

8. There is a potential risk of an expanding haematoma in the spinal canal and possible compression of the spinal cord or nerves after lumbar puncture in patients with blood clotting disorders or on anticoagulants.

Solutions for spinal subarachnoid anaesthesia can be 'hypobaric', 'isobaric' or 'hyperbaric', with specific gravities less than, equal to, or greater than CSF (1.007 at body temperature) Hyperbaric solutions (local anaesthetics mixed with 5 to 10% glucose) are commonly used because their spread can be increased or limited by tilting the patient 'head down' or 'head up' immediately after injection. The hyperbaric solution most commonly used in the United Kingdom is 'heavy' bupivacaine 0.5% of which 2 to 3 ml are usually required. Isobaric 0.5% bupivacaine, as supplied in ordinary ampoules for other local anaesthetic purposes, also enjoys some popularity at the present time — before the solution becomes 'fixed' it can be imagined (so far as adjusting the extent of the block is concerned) as behaving like the bubble in a spirit level. The use of hypobaric solutions has been discontinued — largely because of the unpredictability of the upward spread.

Technique of spinal subarachnoid anaesthesia. The main points have already been considered or implied: preloading with 500–1000 ml of colloid or electrolyte intravenous fluids, a meticulous sterile technique with sterile equipment, careful positioning of the patient with the patients' spine curved to widen the gaps between the vertebrae. After infiltration of the skin, subcutaneous tissues and the interspinous ligament at L2/3 or L3/4 level with local anaesthetic solution, lumbar puncture is performed.

The slope of the table is adjusted after the hyperbaric solution is injected into the CSF. The onset of the block is fairly rapid but at least 10 min should be allowed before permitting surgery to start. Patients injected with small volumes of hyperbaric solutions while sitting, and kept in that position for 5–10 min, will develop a block confined to the perineum ('saddle block'). This is useful for vaginal or rectal procedures.

Lumbar and thoracic epidural anaesthesia

The indications and popularity of this technique for the relief of pain in spontaneous and instrumental vaginal delivery and for caesarean section are increasing; and the use of the technique for transurethral urological operations, particularly in elderly and frail patients, is also once again becoming popular.

Advantages and disadvantages of epidural block compared to subarachnoid block

Advantages

1. It is usually easier to gauge and limit the extent of the spread of an epidural because the contents of the epidural space are not fluid. The insertion of an epidural catheter makes it possible to 'build up' the required dose and repeat it[1].
2. Since the dura is not punctured, the dangers of meningitis, postanaesthetic headache and damage to the spinal cord are reduced.

Disadvantages

1. The epidural block may be patchy due to anatomical variations, e.g. fibrous septa in the epidural space.
2. Much larger doses of local anaesthesia are required for epidural than for spinal subarachnoid anaesthesia. Blood levels can be high, and this can lead to impairment of cardiac function and reduction in cardiac output in elderly patients with an imperfect myocardium.
3. The technique of placing the point of the epidural needle in the epidural space and of feeding a catheter through it (see below) is more exacting than the lumbar puncture required for spinal subarachnoid anaesthesia. The signs of the correct placing of the needle tip are also less definite than CSF aspiration. The failure rate, at least in the hands of the occasional user or beginner, is therefore greater with the epidural than with the subarachnoid technique.
4. There is always the danger that either the needle or the catheter may enter a vessel and systemic injecton will therefore cause profound hypotension.
5. It is also possible that the dura will be penetrated with the

---

[1] The practice of placing catheters in the subarachnoid space for incremental techniques has largely been abandoned because of the dangers of infection and neurological damage.

wide bore needle required for catheterisation causing a high incidence of spinal headache due to leakage of CSF.

6. If the dura is penetrated accidentally, but not detected, a volume of local anaesthetic several times that required for subarachnoid spinal anaesthesia may be injected causing a 'total' spinal with hypotension, unconsciousness and apnoea.

Meticulous attention to the details of the technique and careful testing will reduce the likelihood of these complications, but they may happen even in the hands of experts.

Sympathetic blockade occurs with both epidural and subarachnoid blocks, can cause dangerous hypotension in the presence of hypovolaemia and must be countered by posture and intravenous fluid.

The reliability of pain relief for cutting surgery in the conscious patient is much less with epidurals than with subarachnoid spinals.

Technique of lumbar epidural block. The procedure and precautions are as described above for spinal subarachnoid block up to the point where the needle penetrates the skin at the desired level.

The needle is advanced into the interspinous ligament until it is gripped by it. A syringe containing either air or saline is then attached to the hub of the needle and pressure is applied to the plunger. Resistance will be felt to the injection of the air or saline[2].

The needle is advanced with pressure on the plunger, either continuously or intermittently, until the tip of the needle emerges from the thicker part of the interspinous ligament (the ligamentum flavum) into the epidural space, when there will be an immediate loss of resistance and the air or saline can be injected freely. The width of the epidural space

---

[2] Endless arguments continue among the experts whether air or saline is best. It is not for us to rehearse them here.

is only 0.5 cm, so that great care must be taken to avoid penetration of the dura.

If a one-shot epidural is to be administered, local anaesthetic solution may now be injected. A special wide bore needle (the Tuohy needle) is used if a catheter is to be introduced — Tuohy needles have an ingenious curved tip to direct the catheter in the space. In either case a small test dose is given to ensure that the needle tip has not entered the subarachnoid space. This would be apparent from rapid onset of block and decreased blood pressure.

The position of the patient and gravity have only marginal influence on the spread of the solution because the contents of the epidural space are not fluid like the CSF. The number of segments affected by the local anaesthetic varies with a number of factors: such as, whether the veins in the epidural space are dilated and occupy more space (as in pregnancy) or whether the intervertebral foramina are closed and solution spread into the paravertebral spaces is prevented (as in old age) — in both of these cases a given volume will spread over more segments. The volume required to anaesthetise 4 segments on either side of the needle point in the adult is 12 to 16 ml (1.5–2 ml per segment) — with such a wide variation it is obviously advantageous to 'build up' the spread of the solution by incremental injection through a catheter.

Thoracic epidural block is a more difficult technique because of the obliquity of the spines and the additional potential danger that penetration through the dura might damage the spinal cord itself. Thoracic epidural block with a catheter has special application in the control of pain from thoracic trauma and after major thoracic and abdominal surgery. Careful monitoring and fluid replacement is required and the patients are best managed in an intensive care or high dependency nursing unit.

Caudal block is a useful and effective technique for operations and procedures around the perineum. Occasional users and beginners may have difficulty in locating the sacral hiatus. Once this has been accomplished accurately the insertion of the needle is usually not difficult, even though its angulation has to be changed when the sacrococcygeal membrane is penetrated. The caudal epidural space is quite large and the dural sac ends at S2, so that penetration of the dura is unlikely. Careful aspiration tests should be performed because of the large plexus of veins in the caudal space.

The lumbar epidural space is, of course, a continuation of the caudal space. If sufficient volume of local analgesic is injected it will spread up into the lumbar space and can be used to anaesthetise the legs and upper abdomen. There is, however, a limit to the amount that can be injected in this way before toxic levels are reached. The volumes required are greater per segment in the sacral region (3–4 ml per segment — 20 ml to anaesthetise all 5 sacral segments).

Paravertebral block is included here because of its connection with the epidural space through the intervertebral foramina. It is useful for providing analgesia for unilateral operations such as those on the gall bladder, a single kidney or a thoracotomy. The connection of the spaces with the epidural space must be remembered, since unwanted and wider effects than those intended, including bilateral spread, occur from time to time.

The injection of narcotic analgesics into the subarachnoid and epidural spaces

In the last 10 years it has been shown that not only are there receptors for morphine-like drugs in the spinal cord and brain, but that morphine-like compounds are produced in those regions. The endogenous agents, (enkephalins) are secreted in response to painful stress, and possibly act presynaptically to block the release of the neurotransmitters.

Some of the naturally occurring enkephalins were used to

reduce pain by injecting them into the subarachnoid or epidural spaces. The logical progression is to use opiates in the same way.

Almost every available analgesic has now been injected into the CSF or epidural space. The result has been to discover that the quality of pain relief is less than that produced by conventional local anaesthetic drugs, but the duration is longer and motor block does not result. Side effects such as itching, urinary retention, nausea and vomiting are fairly common, especially following morphine itself. Central respiratory depression is insidious, potentially fatal, and thought to be delayed by the slow absorption and gradual onset of systemic effects of subarachnoid or extradural opiates. Naloxone is rapid and effective treatment, but it is probably best give repeatedly because of its short action.

It is wise to use spinal and epidural narcotics only where surveillance of the patient's respiration can be continued up to 24 h, and any respiratory depression rapidly treated. There would be immense potential for improved analgesic drugs to be given by these routes, particularly if their action is only on specific pain pathways, thus sparing the patients from motor block or other side effects.

10

Anaesthesia for the surgical specialties

'An expert is a man who comes from afar, bearing slides'.
Michael O'Donnell (born 1928)

The days are gone when *any* doctor or dentist was expected to be able to give a competent anaesthetic for *any* operation but, nonetheless, until recent times the anaesthetist has regarded himself as a generalist able to provide anaesthetic care for any type of surgery. This is no longer the case so far as some branches of specialist surgery are concerned, and anaesthetists in large hospitals tend to specialise so that patients in every branch of surgery can enjoy optimum care.

Neonatal surgery

Most anaesthetists expect to manage older children for routine surgery, but there is an increasing tendency to regard the administration of anaesthesia to neonates (0–3 months) and infants (3–12 months) as the province of the specialist. Whenever possible they should be sent to a specialist unit, monitored and resuscitated *en route*, rather than be allowed to satisfy the ambitions of unpractised surgical teams, with inadequate nursing staff left literally holding the baby.

Neonates and infants cannot be regarded as small adults. It is not enough simply to adjust the dosage of drugs, ventilation and gas requirements in proportion to body weight. The neonate has a number of peculiarities:

1. The ductus arteriosus and the foramina in the interatrial and interventricular septa do not close for some days after birth.
2. Fetal haemoglobin has a high affinity for oxygen and may not be totally replaced by adult haemoglobin for several weeks.
3. The central nervous system, renal and hepatic function, the temperature regulating system, and some drug metabolising systems may not mature until the infant is several weeks old. Neonates are sensitive to competitive muscle relaxants but resistant to depolarising agents.
4. The lungs are more easily damaged by excessive ventilatory pressure, causing a pneumothorax or pneumomediastinum.
5. The high metabolic rate results in a far smaller reserve of oxygen; and so the lack of a suffcient concentration of oxygen in inspired gases causes dangerous hypoxia faster than in adults. The neonate does seem to withstand the insult of hypoxia better than older children and adults, but this is no reason to expose a neonate (or anyone else) to hypoxia.
6. Access to the circulation and airway may be difficult and neonates may be difficult to monitor — not least because of the swarm of onlookers that seem to be readily attracted.

Premedication should be an antisialagogue (atropine 0.1–0.2 mg) to reduce coughing and secretions. The use of opioid analgesics pre- or postoperatively is controversial in neonates and the newborn. The risk of respiratory depression means that proportionately half sized doses should be used based on body weight and close observation with intubation facilites is necessary.

Induction Many paediatric anaesthetists, skilled as they are at entering tiny veins, prefer intravenous induction (thiopentone 3–5 mg/kg). Others use inhalation induction with oxygen rich mixtures with or without nitrous oxide. Halothane is less irritant to the airway than isoflurane. Enflurane is effective but less potent and higher concentrations must be used. Cyclopropane 50% in oxygen is still popular in certain centres but is potentially explosive, and therefore often not readily available.

Intubation. Anaesthesia before intubation may not be necessary for children of less than 5 kg body weight and may be hazardous. The risk of stridor is enhanced by mucosal swelling in small airways from irritation of the larynx by the tube, instruments or vapours. Uncuffed tubes small enough to allow a leak of gases should be used. A throat pack will stop fluids passing the tube and entering the lungs. Small infants of less than 5 kg body weight cannot sustain spontaneous respiration well through narrow tracheal tubes and should be ventilated[1].

Apparatus with minimal dead space and low resistance such as the Jackson Rees T-piece (Chapter 7) should be used. Neonates must be kept warm because of their large surface area in proportion to their mass, their undeveloped temperature regulating systems, and poor insulating body fat. The theatre should be at least 22°C (75°F), blankets and warmed mattresses used, intravenous fluids should be warmed and temperature probes inserted into rectum or pharynx.

The management of older children

The principles set out above for neonates apply, but less

[1] This philosophy is admirably summed up by a well known American paediatric anesthesiologist who advises 'PTS' = 'Paralyse the sucker' or 'infants still being fed from bottle or breast should be ventilated'.

emphatically, as children get older. The temperature of the theatre can be more tolerable, but that of the patient must be carefully monitored and managed.

Premedication for the older child is a subject hotly debated over many years. Children between 1 year and about 7 years can become distressed and suffer psychological trauma but they are not always able to comprehend reasoned explanation. Over 7 years (the traditional 'age of reason') most children will listen to an explanation, and provided they are not in pain, it is probably best for them to be aware that they are being taken to the operating theatre and why. Scaled down adult premedications such as traditional intramuscular 'omnopon and scopolamine' for the emergencies, or elixirs of benzodiazepines such as diazepam are often appropriate.

The 'under-sevens' remain a problem. Much depends on the way that they are handled by the whole medical and nursing team; a difficult combination of kindness and firmness is required. Drugs can play only a supporting role. Some paediatric anaesthetists believe that, given the proper nursing environment and attitudes, most small children scheduled for elective surgery are best allowed to play unpremedicated until the time for them to be taken by their mother into a suitably furnished anaesthetic room. The traditional heavy barbiturate premedication given rectally or orally by 'tricking' the pain-free child into an oblivion from which he wakes in agony can result in psychological trauma — but sometimes with a difficult child, it is the lesser evil. The ideal for elective surgery in this age group would probably be a tranquilizer which would render the child dreamily aware that something is happening. Oral trimeprazine (3–4 mg/kg) goes some way towards this ideal, but patients are sometimes disorientated and dysphoric, though amnesic, in the anaesthetic room, especially when subjected to an inhalation induction. The combination of oral trimeprazine (3 mg/kg) with a minimal dose of an intramuscular narcotic (pethidine 1 mg/kg or morphia

0.2 mg/kg) after the former has taken its effect has been found to mitigate dysphoria. Antisialagogues are usually desirable (atropine 0.02 mg/kg) especially if mask anaesthesia is to be used, except for the pyrexial patient. Atropine may be administered orally in about twice the dose used intramuscularly. Emergency cases over 1 year of age (10 kg), particularly those in pain, are best given an intramuscular narcotic (morphia 0.15 mg/kg or omnopon 0.3 mg/kg) with atropine (0.02 mg per kg) or scopolamine (0.006 mg/kg).

Intravenous induction. The same drugs may be used for intravenous induction as for adults. Great care must be taken to ensure that the cannula or needle is in the vein — a child cannot distinguish the particular pain of an extravenous injection from the assault of the whole proceedings. The infusion system should be flushed through between injections. It may contain amounts of drugs which would have a significant effect on the small child.

Use thiopentone (3–5 mg/kg) or methohexitone (1.5 mg/kg). Ketamine is more favoured than in adults, as children appear not to mind the hallucinations which often accompany its use, or not to suffer such bad dreams as adults. Ketamine (1–2 mg/kg intravenously) is less irritant than thiopentone and other induction agents and it is, therefore, safer to use if there is doubt that a needle or cannula is in the vein. Ketamine is also valuable as an induction agent when given intramuscularly (4–8 mg/kg), particularly if veins are nonexistent or the child is not cooperative. The use of ketamine orally and rectally as an analgesic for changing surgical dressings and other purposes is being investigated and shows promise.

[2] One of the authors was convinced that the preliminary chatting up of the diminutive four-year-old outpatient had achieved perfect cooperation, but in the short time it took to be diverted briefly while simply reaching for the mask, the child had slipped through his grasp, jumped off the chair and escaped through the door.

Inhalation induction allows the anaesthetist to show off his skills but the result can vary from almost an artistic performance to a near shambles.[2]

A parent should accompany the child to the anaesthetic room, with the option of staying or returning to the ward. Much influences this decision; if good rapport has been achieved previously between the child and anaesthetist many parents embrace the opportunity to help with the induction, but some will feel relieved at not being obliged to have the experience of seeing their child lose consciousness; it should usually be the parent's choice if the anaesthetist is comfortable with the situation.

The child should be cuddled by the parent or nurse while monitoring is established; electrocardiogram electrodes are easily applied to the child's back without distress and yield valuable information about heart rate and rhythm.

The anaesthetist must have total control during an inhalational induction. The door should be locked; only the parent, one anaesthetic nurse and perhaps one other helper should be present. It is not the right time for the surgeon to remind himself upon which part of the anatomy he is to operate.

The gases flow over the child's face, using the cupped hand as a mask to begin with. The least irritant and most pleasant combination to start is nitrous oxide with oxygen (70/30). The anaesthetist alone should do the talking, as this makes it easier to 'talk' the mask onto the face while encouraging the child to breathe deeply.

Before an airtight fit between mask and face is attained, the child breathes ambient air with the medical gases. The consequent dilution of the anaesthetic mixture causes a longer induction and the child thus has a greater chance of devising method of escape. Reluctant schoolchildren respond well to being firmly told that 'they must just stay there and get on with breathing in and out'. Induction of difficult younger patients should be hastened by the bold addition of halothane. It is fortunate that repeated halothane anaesthetics do not seem to carry even a small risk of hepatitis for children under 8 years.

If the child accepts the anaesthetic peacefully, 0.25% halothane should be given until the child is accustomed to the smell; then it is increased by 0.5% every four good breaths until surgical anaesthesia is achieved with 2 to 4%. An intravenous needle can then be inserted with the child unresponsive, breathing safely and vasodilated. This is a good time for the parent to leave.

With practice, induction can be rapidly achieved under 2 min — very different from smothering techniques of former days. Uncooperative children can rarely be deceived into 'blowing up the football' or 'smelling the scent' — television has brought reality to all but the smallest.

The anaesthetist must then decide between mask anaesthesia and intubation. The latter can be achieved with or without the aid of muscle relaxants. With small children, or if there are airway abnormalities, it is safest to deepen anaesthesia until a tube can be inserted while spontaneous respiration continues. If there is doubt about the ability of a clear airway to be secured by passing a tube, the anaesthetist must demonstrate that he can ventilate the lungs using the bag and mask before committing the patient to paralysis from muscle relaxants.

Smaller laryngoscope blades are used for children, the type depending on anaesthetist's preference and any airway abnormality. Tracheal tubes are chosen on the principle that *cuffed* tubes are not used under size 7, and the next two lower should be ready for immediate use. The narrowest place in the air passage is below the vocal cords in the child.

Emergence and recovery for children can be as terrifying as induction. Parents should be encouraged to be with the child. Adequate analgesia must be given. For minor surgery paracetamol elixir (120 mg in 5 ml) is satisfactory (3 m to 1 year 2.5–5 ml; 1–6 years 5–10 ml; 6–12 years 10–20 ml) or the same doses can be given in rectal suppository form. Intramuscular analgesia with narcotic drugs may be necessary (e.g., morphine 0.1–0.2 mg/kg), but not in infants under 5 kg for risk of respiratory depression, for whom codeine phosphate 1 mg/kg is preferred. If maintainence is with spontaneous respiration and it is anticipated that there will be postoperative pain, an intramuscular injection of narcotic analgesic can be given during the anaesthetic.

Laryngospasm is common after surgery in infants and responds to oxygen and humidification. Temperature fall must be prevented by warmed blankets. Local analgesia can reduce postoperative discomfort, — e.g. caudal block for circumcision.

Local anaesthesia for conscious children is contrary to tradition in the United Kingdom but in many countries it is practised successfully covered by tranquillizing sedation as with minimal doses of oral diazepam.

Obstetric anaesthesia, and analgesia

Obstetrics is a controversial subject and so are the accompanying anaesthetic and analgesic techniques. Where the two meet there has been traditionally a lively disagreement. Although prejudices persist, obstetricians and midwives have gradually accepted the value of the contribution of the anaesthetist in providing pain relief for labour and operative delivery. Anaesthesia for caesarean sections and improvements in local and general techniques for operative delivery have been encouraged by self scrutiny by all involved in obstetric care. This has been prompted by the publication of national reports in Britain every 3 years of the causes of maternal mortality — a unique attempt to analyse mishaps in care, and to define where they can be rectified.

General anaesthesia. The principal cause of anaesthetic related death remains aspiration of stomach contents. Pregnant women, especially when in labour, are particularly at risk when they present as emergencies — often after a recent meal. Gastric emptying is delayed in pregnancy or labour and by narcotic drugs, and thus there is often a greater residue of stomach contents than in the conventional surgical patient.

The acidity of the stomach contents is also abnormally high during pregnancy and consequently, if aspiration occurs, serious damage to the lung can be caused. The condition known as Mendelson's syndrome is characterised by tight bronchospasm, hypoxia and collapse of the alveoli due to the bronchospasm, hypoxia, and destruction of surfactant (the lipoprotein which reduces surface tension and keeps them open) causing severe pulmonary damage. The condition may fail to respond to intermittent positive pressure ventilation, oxygen, steroids, antibiotics and all the conventional methods of managing respiratory failure. The tragedy is compounded by the victim usually being a fit, healthy young woman expecting an uncomplicated delivery. Despite many attempts to reduce the hazards, Mendelson's syndrome continues to claim lives.

The prophylactic measures which can be taken to avoid such a tragedy are fully discussed in Chapter 11. Patients in labour who are known to be liable to require surgical intervention should be starved, and hydrated by intravenous infusion if necessary. It is not the usual practice to pass oro- or nasogastric tubes before obstetric surgery.

Cricoid pressure should be used during tracheal intubation. The oesophagus can effectively be occluded during the time of the greatest risk of regurgitation by firm digital pressure applied directly backward on the cricoid cartilage (Sellick's manoeuvre). The pressure should be maintained until the airway is secured by the cuffed tracheal tube, and an airtight seal has been demonstrated. A trained assistant is necessary.

A tipping patient trolley should be used during induction and the anaesthetist must ensure that suction apparatus is to hand and working.

Another potential hazard is supine hypotension. The gravid uterus obstructs the inferior vena cava and aorta if the patient lies flat on her back. If the patient is tilted to one side, preferably to the left, the condition can be relieved.

A sequence of preoxygenation, Sellick's manoeuvre, intravenous thiopentone 4 mg/kg suxamethonium 1 mg/kg, tracheal intubation, ventilation with N_2O/O_2 50% mixture with added 0.5% halothane, and tubocurarine 0.5 mg/kg, is satisfactory in most cases. Immediately after the delivery of the infant, the mother is given intravenous analgesia (papaveretum 10–20 mg) is given.

There is growing tendency for the use of regional anaesthetic techniques in operative delivery. Pudendal nerve block is widely used for forceps delivery. The use of subarachnoid spinal or epidural block (see below) avoids the risks of general anaesthesia. The mother, who is conscious, can protect her own airway during the delivery. The all important bonding between mother and child is also promoted if the mother does not awaken to be faced by an unknown infant which she can only presume to be hers.

The placental barrier. One of the major concerns of anaesthetists is whether the drugs which they use may cross the placental barrier and harm the fetus. The principal factors governing transfer are low molecular weight (if it is over 600, transfer is likely to be very slow); lipid solubility (drugs must be lipid soluble to enter cell lipid membranes to cross the placental barrier); and whether the particular drug is ionised (positively-charged ionised drugs are repelled by the charge on cell membranes and are thus less likely to cross it readily). Other less important factors are: the dose of the drug and the rapidity of injection; the site of administration of the drug (the closer the drug is injected to the uterine artery the less it will be diluted and the greater the concentration effect).

Uterine contraction causes a massive increase in intra-uterine pressure which often exceeds the perfusion pressure. No drug transfer occurs while there is this temporary cessation of perfusion. Canny anaesthetists inject drugs like thiopentone to coincide with a uterine contraction and thus gain maximal benefit from this effect.

Transfer of anaesthetic drugs matters particularly in early pregnancy up to 12 weeks (when there is a risk of inducing fetal abnormalities or an abortion) and at term when depression of the fetal central nervous system and neonatal respiration can result.

Obstetric analgesia. The available techniques for the relief of pain in normal vaginal delivery vary from the nonpharmacological to the relatively invasive technique of continuous epidural blockade. They include:-

1. *'Natural' techniques* involving careful and extensive antenatal education in relaxation.
2. *Hypnosis.* This avoids the use of drugs but success depends on a combination of the patient's susceptibility, time spent in preparation and the hypnotists's skill. The technique is most successful on a one-to-one basis but self hypnosis can be taught to suitable subjects.
3. *Acupuncture* and transcutaneous nerve stimulation. No drugs to depress the fetus are given but the technique requires a suitable receptive patient, skill and confidence in its use and in placing, manipulating and managing the acupuncture needles.
4. *Inhalational analgesia* originated with chloroform used for pain relief in childbirth by James Young Simpson, Professor of Obstetrics in Edinburgh in 1847. The commonest technique in the United Kingdom today is the use of premixed nitrous oxide and oxygen (Entonox®, 50%, nitrous oxide and 50% oxygen). This is a useful method of providing analgesia accompanied by a high concentration

of oxygen, with rapid onset and cessation, and minimal (if any) adverse effects on the infant. The mother holds the mask herself, so that if she becomes too drowsy it falls away from her face; she thus has considerable control over the administration. The method does not provide complete freedom from pain however, and may be inadequate for prolonged or particularly painful labours; it also encourages hyperventilation. Attempts to improve analgesia by holding the mask on the face of the patient are ill advised; undue depth of anaesthesia may result. Trichloroethylene, enflurane and isoflurane have also been used.

5. *Injected analgesia*. The midwife is the only member of the nursing profession in the United Kingdom who is authorised to prescribe and administer narcotic drugs on her own initiative. The drug most frequently chosen is pethidine (meperidine, U.S.) and two 100 mg doses can be given by an unsupervised midwife. Pethidine produces useful pain relief in many patients, but only rarely completely abolishes the pain of contractions. Pethidine is most useful if it is administered in time to cover the later part of the second stage of labour. It is a potent respiratory depressant and is frequently associated with depression of breathing in the newborn up to 6 h after the last administration. The intramuscular injection of naloxone (0.2 mg) administered to the newborn infant reduces the hazard but may have a shorter effect than the pethidine; respiratory depression may therefore return and the naloxone have to be repeated.

6. *Epidural analgesia*. One of the greatest areas of expansion in anaesthetic practice has been obstetric pain relief by continuous epidural block. This followed the introduction of effective bacterial filters, improved methods of sterilization of drugs and apparatus, the production of freely available packs of sterile equipment, needles, etc., and the introduction of bupivacaine (Marcain). Bupivacaine is a

long acting local anaesthetic. It can produce 2–6 h of pain relief, and has much less effect on the motor power of the muscles responsible for expulsion of the fetus than most other anaesthetic agents. The newborn infant is unlikely to be impaired by the technique of the drugs, providing the maternal blood pressure is not allowed to fall from sympathetic blockade.

The success of continuous lumbar epidural blocks depends upon understanding of the pain pathways during labour and delivery. The pain of the first stage is conveyed through the posterior roots of the 10th, 11th, 12th, thoracic nerves and the 1st lumbar nerves. Thus block of these segments by local anaesthetuc solution instilled into the epidural space will cause reduction or abolition of the pain of early labour. Ideally pain is relieved while other sensations, like pressure, are retained. The mother can still appreciate being in labour without either being in pain or incapable of feeling some of its sensations.

In some units, anaesthetists elect to administer the 'top up' doses of local analgesic, but in others midwives are trained to do so. Rarely, the level of the epidural may become so high that the respiratory nerves are blocked and immediate resuscitation and artificial ventilation are necessary. Despite this risk, the mishaps from regional techniques are few and usually trivial. A continuous epidural block given through an indwelling cannula can be extended or adjusted to cover caesarean section without recourse to general anaesthesia.

The advantages and disadvantages of epidurals in obstetrics.
The advantages include :-
1. The avoidance of narcotic drugs, thus reducing the possibilities of prolonged respiratory and central nervous
   depression of the infant and vomiting in the mother.
2. Complete analgesia is possible.

3. The block can be adjusted to provide adequate analgesia for operative delivery in caesarean section.
4. The mother's consciousness remains unclouded throughout.
5. After delivery, analgesia can be adequate for suturing, removal of retained placenta, etc.
6. Blood loss is reduced.
7. Changes in maternal, and consequental fetal, acid–base state are minimal, since hyperventilation and acidosis are reduced.
8. An indwelling epidural cannula can be used to administer epidural narcotics after operative delivery, provided close observation of respiration is maintained.

The disadvantages are:-
1. Restriction of the mobility of the mother.
2. Risk of decrease in maternal blood pressure from a combination of peripheral vasodilation in the lower part of the body (from sympathetic blockade), and obstruction of the vena cava and/or the aorta when the uterus falls backwards, if the mother is in the supine position. All patients who are to have regional blockade in labour should first be given a fluid load by an intravenous infusion of crystalloid solution (Hartmann's 500 ml). This fills up the expanded intravascular space caused by the increase in diameter of the blood vessels when the vasoconstrictor sympathetic nerve plexuses are blocked. An essential precaution is to tilt the patient to one side, so that the pressure from the weighty uterus does not fall directly on to the major blood vessels. The patient should have been asked whether she felt faint during late pregnancy if lying in a supine position. It will inevitably follow that such patients will develop profound hypotension if they are not tilted laterally in the supine position after an epidural block. Resuscitation facilities must be to hand for ventilating with 100% oxygen, intravenous vasoconstrictor

drugs (ephedrine up to 30 mg in 5 mg doses) and a tilting bed must be available to enable the mother to be put head down.

3. Outlet forceps deliveries are probably more common after epidural block because the mother may be less able to push effectively during the second stage; but epidural blocks are indicated for patients who already have complicated labours requiring early assistance to shorten the second stage and prevent undue deterioration in the condition of the fetus.

4. Other side effects are backache, urinary retention, and shivering.

5. Rarely, adverse effects from accidental dural puncture result, as headache. Excessive subarachnoid spread of the block may occur if the error is not recognised, and a full epidural dose of local anaesthetic is injected through a needle advanced too far during insertion.

Caudal analgesia may also be used. It is valuable for perineal pain, but requires greater volumes of solution than a lumbar epidural block with increased risk of fetal depression.

Spinal blocks have been employed for many years for surgical delivery, but only recently has it become easy, with improved sterility and drugs, to offer them to patients in labour.

Gynaecological surgery

The scope of gynaecological surgery is obviously limited by gender and by being confined to the lower part of the abdomen or perineum.[3]

---

[3] An anaesthetist was heard to admonish his gynaecological colleagues with the accusation that they only carry out four operations and all on one organ. They are confined to, *looking* (laparoscopy), *scraping* (D & C) evacuations and terminations, *hitching* (anterior or posterior repairs and colposuspension) and *removing* (vaginal and abdominal hysterectomy). As a refinement, irradiation is used to combat tumours.

There are some particular problems. Females tend to vomit postoperatively more than males, especially if undergoing surgery which involves stretching the cervix; and drugs may be required which are also potent emetic agents (for example ergometrine, or prostaglandin pessaries, given before vaginal termination of pregnancy or for retained products of conception).

Spinal, lumbar epidural or caudal blocks, whether or not accompanied by sedation or general anaesthesia, are admirable for gynaecological procedures because they reduce the incidence of postoperative deep vein thrombosis, bleeding and ileus. The patient can also enjoy postoperative pain relief without the adverse effects of narcotic analgesics.

The pregnant uterus contracts less efficiently when exposed to the halogenated anaesthetic agents, this discourages the use of halothane, enflurane or isoflurane for evacuation of retained products of conception. The problems which derive from inadequate anaesthesia when those agents are not used are possibly greater than the potential hazard of excessive blood loss during a brief anaesthetic. Halothane 0.5%, isoflurane 0.75% or enflurane 1.0% are acceptable maintenance concentrations, and higher concentrations can be used during induction, but intermittent thiopentone or propofol with fentanyl or alfentanil and nitrous oxide and oxygen is a satisfactory alternative technique.

Neurosurgery

The problems of anaesthesia for neurosurgery stem from the brain being enclosed within a rigid box. Any change in the volume of the contents of the cranium will cause a change of the pressure within, and alteration in the perfusion of the brain. The factors which affect the intracranial pressure, apart from space occupying lesions (tumours. haemorrhage, etc.) are the size and distension of the blood vessels and the volume of cerebrospinal fluid.

The brain perfusion is maintained over a greater range of blood pressure than any other organ, but alterations in the blood pressure or calibre of the blood vessels frequently result from anaesthetic drugs and techniques. Cerebral blood vessels are dilated by the volatile inhalational agents (halothane, enflurane and isoflurane), by an increase in arterial carbon dioxide (which may result from hypoventilation) and if vasodilator drugs (nitroprusside, nitroglycerine or ganglion blockers) are used.

Veins may become distended in the brain by occlusion of their outflow through obstruction in the neck, or through raised central venous pressure from other causes (coughing and straining, positive pressure ventilation, congestive heart failure, overtransfusion, etc.) or may distend by hypercarbia or hypoxia.

The perfusion pressure of the brain is the resultant of the difference between arterial and venous pressures, minus intracranial pressure (ICP). The anaesthetist must attempt to avoid an increase in the ICP, especially if it is already raised by a tumour, clot or carbon dioxide retention. The increase in ICP, which would otherwise accompany the use of the volatile agents, can be counteracted by hyperventilation and this can be achieved most easily after tracheal intubation. Laryngoscopy and insertion of the tube also may raise intracranial pressure and must be minimised by the liberal use of narcotic analgesics, topical anaesthesia and an adequate dose of intravenous induction agent; beta-blocking agents have also been used.

Intra-operative problems for the neuroanaesthetist include the possibility of air embolism, this may occur if large veins are opened to the atmosphere during posterior fossa explorations with the patient in the sitting position); haemorrhage from poorly contracted cerebral vessels; and difficulty of access to the airway while surgery is in progress.

Other methods, which may be used by the anaesthetist to reduce intracranial pressure both during the operation and postoperatively include the use of osmotic diuretics (mannitol 20% 0.5 mg/kg body weight, intravenously to increase fluid loss and decrease cerebrospinal fluid (CSF) volume and production), and the drainage of CSF through a fine needle inserted into the spinal canal in the lumbar region. Dexamethasone (8 to 20 mg) is also used to reduce cerebral oedema by stabilising cell membranes and thus reduces their permeability after an hypoxic or traumatic insult.

Eye surgery

Eye surgeons have the smallest anatomical area of specialisation and there are special anaesthetic considerations. Many elderly eye patients suffer from a variety of cardiac and pulmonary diseases, and diabetes is a special problem. It is fortunate, therefore, that a number of ophthalmological operations can be carried out under local anaesthesia, including cataract extraction in the elderly, one of the most frequent procedures. Special knowledge and expertise is required if general anaesthesia is necessary either because of the temperament of the patient or the nature or length of the procedure (modern operations for detached retina for example).

Intraocular procedures. The anaesthetist must tailor his anaesthetic to avoid a rise in and, if possible, to reduce intraocular pressure. If pressure rises when the eye is open, whether surgically or from a penetrating wound, the vitreous will be extruded — like the contents of a grape when it is squeezed, and the sight of the eye may be lost. A number of factors will cause a rise in intraocular pressure (IOP) if not counteracted; these include straining, coughing, and vomiting (which engorge the veins within the eye), increases in blood pressure (which causes more aqueous humour to be produced) and contraction of the extraocular muscles. Suxamethonium causes a contraction of the extraocular muscles which squeezes the eye. If the eye is closed IOP will subside after intubation when the effect of the suxamethonium wears off, but if the eye is already open, as with a penetrating wound, vitreous is squeezed out with disastrous consequences.

The art of giving anaesthesia for eye surgery thus entails giving adequate doses of induction agent and muscle relaxants to avoid hypertension and prevent extraocular muscle contraction, adequate use of local anaesthetics on the larynx to avoid straining and hypertension at intubation, and the use of antiemetics to avoid vomiting. Furthermore, surgeons should never be discouraged from combining local blocks around the eye with general anaesthesia.

Extraocular procedures. Squint surgery is the most common in this category. The main hazards are reflexes initiated on traction on the extraocular muscles mediated by the vagus nerve if the patient is too deeply anaesthetised. These reflexes are: the oculocardiac reflex causing bradycardia; the oculorespiratory reflex, causing breathholding if the patient is breathing spontaneously; and the oculogastric reflex which may initiate vomiting. The most dangerous of these is the oculocardiac reflex. Adequate anaesthesia and intravenous atropine or glycopyrrolate as preventative measures or as treatment is an answer.

Ear, nose and throat surgery

Tonsillectomy remains the commonest childhood operation and presents challenges for the anaesthetist. The child may have recurrent upper respiratory tract infections and so be liable to postoperative bronchopneumonia. Many children requiring tonsillectomy have impaired hearing too and, until grommets are inserted, communication may be impaired. Enlarged, chronically inflamed tonsils and adenoids may make intubation difficult.

The traditional anaesthetic for tonsillectomy was open drop ether or chloroform given to the child on the kitchen table while intraoral butchery ended in extraction of the afflicted glands. The psychological and/or physical damage to generations of children from such barbaric practices is inestimable. There is still an emotional legacy in the community from such trauma, but the indications for tonsillectomy have been much reduced and the anaesthesia has become less brutal.

Anaesthesia for tonsillectomy differs little in technique from anaesthesia for any major operation. Premedication is necessary to reduce anxiety and secretions; induction can be by inhalation or intravenous means depending on the combined preferences of anaesthetist and child. Intubation is thought nowadays to be necessary for better control over the airway; an oral reinforced or precurved tube is best, which will fit into the slit in the blade of the gag used by the surgeon. An intravenous cannula allows drugs, fluids or blood to be given. A basic principle applying to any operation in the upper airway is that aspiration of blood into the lungs will be much less likely if topical anaesthesia to the larynx is not used. Packs are placed, usually by the surgeon to soak up blood, and pharyngeal suction is used. The child should recover the cough reflex before the tube is removed.

All children should be placed in the 'tonsil position' before extubation while they are still unconscious, (on the side with the under knee bent and the under arm drawn under the body) but this is especially the case after tonsillectomy so that fluid in the upper airway can drain with gravity and be suctioned from the mouth, instead of being drawn into the lungs. *Recovery after tonsillectomy requires the undivided attention of the trained recovery nurse.*

Microscopic middle ear surgery. ENT surgeons have extended their surgical techniques to include microsurgery of the middle ear. This usually requires meticulously conducted anaesthesia to avoid venous congestion and often deliberate hypotension. The simplest technique is to ventilate the patient using halothane, enflurane, or isoflurane and employ a muscle relaxant which promotes hypotension. So great is the magnification of the microscope used by the surgeon that any blood loss looks torrential. Similarly, movement of the operating field by the anaesthetist leaning on the operating table resembles an earthquake.

Tracheostomy is another apparently trivial operation which can be hazardous. It relieves upper airway obstruction, and gains access to the lower respiratory tract for ventilaton or suction. The anaesthetic problems are discussed in the next chapter.

Plastic surgery

Although plastic surgery is confined to operations on the body surface, it includes correction of major congenital defects, microanastomoses of separated blood vessels and nerves in the reimplantation of severed limbs, and the surgical management of burns. Plastic surgery embraces cosmetic surgery, the only specialty in which the reason for surgery may simply be social. Another peculiarity of plastic surgery is that a single operation is often not definitive (for example, scar revision may be required) and this brings the hazards of repeated anaesthesia.

A paradox in plastic surgery anaesthesia is the requirement for dissection of vascular tissues without undue blood loss, yet not to threaten the viability of the tissues either by hypotension or constriction of blood flow to or from the graft when the skin or muscle is replaced in a new position.

Reduction of bleeding is best accomplished by enhancing venous return and raising the operated part of the body above the level of the heart. Reduction of the systemic arterial blood pressure helps and can be achieved by 'tricks' varying frcm a tourniquet to pharmacological manipulation.

Surgeons always expect 'dry' fields without undue bleeding (it speeds the surgery and makes it look artistic) but only in plastic surgery, the surgery of cerebral aneurysms and of the middle ear, is it necessary to provide a totally 'dry' field by profound, deliberate hypotension. Deliberate hypotension is associated with certain risks as it is difficult to affect the systemic circulation without reducing blood flow to the brain and other vital organs; it should be used only by the expert and only when the absence of bleeding is imperative. It should never be employed merely to make a difficult operation easy for a surgeon or to avoid blood transfusion. Safety may be enhanced by electroencephalographic brain monitors.

Modest hypotension (systolic blood pressure 90–100 mmHg) is probably as safe as general anaesthesia. Deliberate induced hypotension with a systolic blood pressure of less than 80 mmHg demands accurate, continuous monitoring with an indwelling arterial cannula and display on a oscilloscope. Hypotension for longer than one hour requires assessment of renal function by continuous collection of urine through a catheter ensuring that at least 0.5 ml/kg/hour is produced.

With the current liberal use of narcotic drugs in general anaesthesia and the preference for intermittent positive pressure ventilation and supplementation of anaesthesia with halothane or isoflurane, there is rarely need for vigorous reduction of blood pressure. Abolition of the hypertensive responses to larnygoscopy and intubation at the beginning of anaesthesia is often the major factor in preventing excessive bleeding.

The techniques which can be used to reduce blood pressure include:-

1. *The tourniquet* which can, of course, only be used for limb surgery. Time is a limiting factor (maximum 90 min for the arm and 120 min for the leg); theoretical disadvantages are tissue damage and metabolic acidosis when tourniquet is released. Tourniquets should not be used for diabetics

or patients with sickle cell trait or disease (Chapter 12), as thrombosis and gangrene may be caused.

2. *Infiltration with vasoconstrictors* (e.g. adrenaline 1:500,000) is usually combined with local anaesthesia but theoretically this is paradoxical, as local anaesthetics are vasodilators. Ventricular dysrythmias may occur especially with halothane, although the risk is less with enflurane or isoflurane. Dosage should be limited and care taken by aspiration and movement of the needle to avoid intravascular injection. Tissue damage and haematoma formation are possible complications.

3. *Reduction in venous pressure* involves the use of posture. The operation site should be uppermost.

4. *A negative phase on the ventilator can be used and venous obstruction should be eliminated.* Hypocarbia produced by hyperventilation will avoid vasodilatation. The disadvantages are that positioning the patient can be awkward and venous air embolism is a possibility, especially with operations on the neck in the head-up position.

5. *Pharmacological reduction of arterial pressure.* Peripheral vascular resistance can be reduced in a number of ways.

   (a) By direct arterial vasodilation, by nitroprusside or nitroglycerine; or the alpha-adrenergic blockers, phenoxybenzamine, phentolamine or droperidol; or by using the halogenated inhalation anaesthetic agents, isoflurane, halothane or enflurane.

   (b) By action on the sympathetic nerve endings by guanethidine, bretylium, or reserpine.

   (c) By blocking sympathetic ganglia in combination with halothane, using trimetaphan or pentolinium.

   (d) By action on muscle blood vessels by, for example, isoflurane.

   There are disadvantages. Vasodilators are potent drugs and may be short acting, the effect may overshoot and produce excessive hypotension, tachyphylaxis is possible and sympathetic nerve ending blockade is altered by pancuronium. Lastly, sympathetic ganglia other than those acting on the arterioles may become blocked, causing ileus and other effects.[4]

6. *Reduction of cardiac output by decreasing the heart rate.* Beta adrenergic blockers, narcotic analgesics and inhalational halogenated anaesthetic agents have this action. The difficulty is that the response to hypovolaemia is abolished, and so recognition and management of surgical bleeding is complicated.

Pulmonary surgery

Preparation. Before any lung operation, pulmonary function tests should establish the state of the lung function and help to predict it after lung tissue is removed. The effects of bronchodilators are also measured, as many patients for pulmonary surgery have an element of treatable bronchoconstriction.[5] Arterial blood gas analysis is also undertaken to indicate the state of gaseous exchange.

[4] In the early days of the use of ganglion blocking agents in the 1950's an anaesthetist had fretted throughout an unexpectedly long hypotensive anaesthetic. He had neither anticipated the duration nor used monitoring as extensively as he would have wished. Both the anaesthetist and the surgeon were greatly alarmed to find that the patient's pupils were huge, fixed and unresponsive. After a few nail-biting hours expecting the patient's brain to be dead, the ganglion blocker wore off, the pupils became responsive and the patient awoke uneventfully. It pays to understand *all* the effects of drugs given during anaesthesia.

[5] One thoracic surgeon preferred his clinical judgement to new fangled function tests and insisted that he, the patient and his registrar all climbed the hospital stairs together. If the patient failed to reach the top of the first flight without breathlessness, he was assessed as unfit for surgery. If he reached the top of two flights, he could withstand a pneumonectomy. When the patient could reach the third floor and the surgeon could not, his registrar was regarded more fit than his consultant to perform the surgery on a particularly healthy patient.

Other preoperative preparation includes physiotherapy to clear retained secretions, breathing exercises to educate the patient for reduced lung volume postoperatively, and chest X-ray to demonstrate the anatomical configuration of the upper respiratory tract.

The pneumothorax problem. As soon a surgical incision or a traumatic wound penetrates the chest wall a pneumothorax is produced. The lung on that side collapses. Severe hypoxia will result which may be fatal, because air oscillates from one lung to another without being properly oxygenated or eliminating carbon dioxide while, at the same time, the mediastinum flaps to and fro. A great deal of effort went into attempts to solve the pneumothorax problem in the first half of the twentieth century. These sometimes involved the construction of massive negative pressure chambers to keep the lung expanded during surgery, but thoracic surgery remained a hazardous undertaking until the introduction of intubation and controlled intermittent positive pressure ventilation, (IPPV) in the 1940's. Double lumen tracheobronchial tubes, (Carlen's, Whites', Bryce-Smith's, Salt's, Robertshaw's etc.), were developed in the 1950's. The tip of these tubes, with the outlet of one lumen, lies in a mainstem bronchus, while the outlet from the other lumen is in the trachea. A seal is formed by inflating a cuff around the tube in each position; each lung can then be isolated and ventilated independently even with an open chest wound. Much early thoracic surgery was applied for the treatment of infection and its consequences (tuberculosis, bronchiectasis, etc.). Endobronchial intubation avoids the danger of contaminated material from the infected operated lung passing into the other and infecting that too.

When only one lung is ventilated, it might seem that half the cardiac output should pass through the collapsed lung and fail to take up oxygen or release carbon dioxide — a 50% shunt would occur — and this would obviously be dangerous.

In practice the situation is not as bad; lung reflexes respond to hypoxia by constricton of the pulmonary vessels, and reduce the blood flow through the collapsed lung. Lateral posture also reduces perfusion of the isolated upper lung which is kept viable by the bronchial circulation.

Premedication should include a drying agent and an analgesic (omnopon and scopolamine are satisfactory). Bronchodilators may be necessary (the use of a salbutamol inhaler for example).

Induction and intubation. After induction of anaesthesia with an intravenous agent and muscle relaxant, preferably while an indwelling arterial line displays arterial blood pressure and gives access for gas analysis, a double-lumen endobronchial tube is passed. These tubes designed with an extra curve on the endobronchial portion are particularly bulky and unwieldy. It demands skill and practice to place them with accuracy. Once the tube is in place, a sequence of inflating the endobronchial and endotracheal cuffs with ventilation of alternate sides of the chest is pursued, until it is certain that the lungs can be separately ventilated and isolated. Intubation of the right main stem bronchus is anatomically easier than the left, as it leaves the trachea at a less acute angle, but the right upper lobe bronchus leaves its main stem bronchus close to the origin, and may be occluded by the tube, unless the specially designed hole is accurately placed at the upper lobe orifice.

After satisfactory intubation has been confirmed, the patient is positioned with the lung to be operated upon uppermost. After the pleura has been opened, ventilation is briefly stopped and the upper lung is allowed to collapse. The lower lung will then be ventilated with the total ventilation which previously went to both lungs. The anaesthetist adjusts the ventilation until the oxygenation and carbon dioxide elimination are satisfactory by blood gas analysis or pulse oximetry. The mediastinum must be kept close to the midline by the inflated lower lung, because if it is allowed to move either upwards or down in the lateral position hypotension will result.

Emergence and recovery. After most chest surgery, a drain is inserted to extract air or blood via a one way valve, (usually a simple underwater seal drain) until any leak is ended. After a pneumonectomy, no drain is inserted but air may be added or removed from the thoracic cavity until the mediastinum is held in the normal position.

At the end of the operation it is often helpful to numb the intercostal nerves supplying the area of the incision and chest drains from within the thorax by injecting a long acting local anaesthetic such as bupivacaine. Alternatively, local anaesthetic may be injected by the surgeon, or the nerves can be frozen with a cryoprobe under direct vision before the chest is closed.

During the recovery phase intermittent positive pressure may be required until the patient can be weaned off the ventilator and breathes for himself.

One-lung anaesthesia may also be used to improve surgical access to other structures in the chest, e.g. the oesophagus, and the same principles apply.

Cardiac surgery

Cardiopulmonary perfusion. In the 1960's machines were developed to assume the basic functions of the heart and lungs. Blood is removed from the venous circulation by gravity or by pump, and passed through heparinised tubing into an oxygenator. After removing any bubbles, the blood is pumped back into the aorta at a pressure sufficient to maintain perfusion around the body. Carbon dioxide is eliminated as the blood passes through the oxygenator, anaesthetic gases or vapours can be added, and the patient's temperature can be exactly controlled by heat exchangers. The blood is no longer circulated through the heart, which can be at a stand-still and emptied. It is infinitely easier to operate on a still, silent heart than on a beating one.

The appearance on cardiopulmonary bypass when the heart is at a standstill, the lungs are silent, the core temperature is a chilly 29°C, the pupils are fixedly dilated, and even the electroencephalogram shows no sign of activity, resembles death as closely as is possible. Yet, when the temperature is allowed to rise, and the heart begins to beat again and is filled with blood, the vital signs gradually return and the patient is restored to life. It is a miracle of Lazarine proportions, but now so commonplace that it is no longer considered remarkable.

The duration of perfusion is limited principally by the effects of the passage of blood through the oxygenator and pumps. Red blood cells become fragmented and break down to release free haemoglobin, which may silt up the kidneys. Air bubbles can enter the systemic circulation and cause embolic damage to the brain, eyes or elsewhere. Bleeding may become a problem, as heparin anticoagulation is necessary to prevent clots being released into the circulation or the oxygenator becoming uselessly filled with clots.

Anaesthetic technique. Although most United Kingdom anaesthetists experience cardiac anaesthesia during their training, few will practice it as consultant, but the skills they have learned are widely useful.

Monitoring techniques for central venous pressure, direct arterial pressure, cardiac output, pulmonary capillary wedge pressure, and experience in the use of potent drugs affecting the heart and circulation has gradually extended into other areas of medicine, particularly coronary care and intensive therapy unit.

Patients must be presented for cardiac surgery with infor-mation from X-rays, cardiac catheterisation, dye and myocar-dial contractility studies, to ensure that the site and extent of the lesion is accurately known and a suitable plan is organised to correct it.

Associated problems include septal defects, shunts from the right to left sides of the heart, dysrhythmias, alterations in blood pressure, myocardial ischaemia, fixed cardiac output, congestive cardiac failure.

1. *Septal defects*. Air or other emboli can pass through a defect between one side of the heart and the other, gain access to the systemic circulation, and lodge in the peripheral circulation. Serious damage is likely if the brain or eye is embolised.

   Shunts of blood from the high-pressure left side of the heart containing oxygenated blood may be reversed if the patient coughs; or strains, or if the extremities become vasoconstricted from cold or drugs. The patient's life may be threatened unless the shunt is surgically corrected or otherwise reversed.

2. *Dysrhythmias*. Some dysrhythmias may be congenital, as in heart block where the conjuction of an atrial impulse fails to reach and trigger ventricular contraction. This is often well tolerated in the young but in later life may require an artificial pacemaker.

   Other dysrhythmias usually result from ischaemic changes or alterations in the normal sequence of impulse, conduction and response. In atrial fibrillation, multiple impulses originating in the atria produce small ineffectual atrial contractions, while the ventricles respond only occasionally or at their own (idioventricular) rate.

   The anaesthetist is faced with the problems of alteration in the normal mechanism of a cardiac output and the likelihood that the drugs used and physiological changes produced by anaesthesia will worsen already impaired cardiac function. There is also the possibility that drugs used to reduce or control the rhythm disturbance may adversely react with the anaesthetic — this will be particularly so when there is electrolyte disturbance, hypovolaemia, altered ventilation or hypoxia or hypercarbia. It is important that the anaesthetist has a good grasp of the patient's problems, and of the anaesthetic factors which may alter or worsen them.

Vascular surgery

Diseased blood vessels can be replaced by grafts to restore circulation in patients previously condemned to suffer ischaemic pain and potential gangrene of the limbs. Vascular surgery techniques also make it possible to operate on blood vessels to remove the obstruction from thrombi, atheromatous plaques or anatomical defects. Many of these patients have a multiplicity of associated problems for the anaesthetist: hypertension, ischaemic heart disease, chronic bronchitis and emphysema are common. If there is no adequate control of a cut blood vessel, or control is lost in the course of surgery, the anaesthetist may have to replace massive losses of blood. It is important to maintain perfusion of threatened tissues by keeping the perfusion pressure high enough without overstimulating the impaired myocardium. The first attempt at surgery on major blood vessels is rarely the last, so the problem of repeated anaesthesia is added.

Invasive monitoring can much improve the management of anaesthesia during major vascular sugery by helping the anaesthetist to balance the loss and replacement of fluid or blood.

Orthopaedic surgery

Patients present for orthopaedic procedures from infancy to advanced old age. Many emergencies are the victims of trauma, and therefore the orthopaedic surgery may be only part of the acute management of their injuries. By contrast, most elective orthopaedic disorders do not threaten life and, consequently, patients may have a lengthy wait for surgery after the decision has been made to operate. The medical problems of such patients may worsen drastically during that delay, and the anaesthetist must be alert to the need for postponing the procedure further until the patient's health is improved.

Most orthopaedic operations, apart from those on the spine, are upon the limbs and therefore suitable for regional or local anaesthetic techniques, particularly as there is little need for muscle relaxation. Similarly, relatively light general anaesthesia can be used without any great necessity for the use of muscle relaxants or intermittent positive pressure ventilation (IPPV) (unless of course the patient has a medical indication for IPPV or is to be operated upon in the face-down position).

The problems which may arise from the use of arterial tourniquets to produce a bloodless surgical field have been discussed earlier in this chapter in connection with plastic surgery.

The hip is one of the commonest orthopaedic operation sites. Hips may require replacement or stabilizing after fracture, and most of these patients are elderly and have widespread osteoporosis. The mortality of fractured hip is high (up to 30% in the first 3 months) but the influence of the anaesthetic in this is difficult to quantify. The choice of anaesthetic technique for correction of fractured hip is controversial. The advantages of prevention of immediate deep venous thrombosis by spinal or other regional anaesthetic techniques may be offset by the potential hazard of hypotension in the elderly. The success of operations under general anaesthesia may, in fact, be due to haemodilution, vasodilation, anticoagulation and other prophylaxis against deep venous thrombosis.

Hip replacement operations have transformed orthopaedic wards over the past 20 years, as the patients no longer spend months in traction. Acute hypotension and cardiovascular collapse when methyl methacrylate cement is pushed into the femoral shaft originally caused great concern, but the dangers of this procedure have reduced. The local substitution of carbon dioxide for air prevents air occupying the hollowed out shaft, and preloading the circulation with intravenous fluids shortly before instillation of the cement is beneficial.

11

Anaesthetists and emergency surgery

> Sign in a Croydon maternity ward: 'The first five minutes of life are the most dangerous.' To which, someone has added: 'The last five minutes are pretty dicey too.'
>
> *The Financial Times.* 1985

The anaesthetist on call should keep in touch with the admission or casualty areas and the wards on take for warning of emergencies. The surgeons will appreciate this early contact and involvement in the patient's preparation. This chapter will illustrate how the patient's surgical condition can affect the conduct of anaesthesia and how the problems can be overcome. The two principal life threatening situations are respiratory obstruction and hypovolaemia. The anaesthetist frequently has to undertake advanced first aid to help the patient survive before anaesthesia for major surgery can be undertaken; the accident situations as well as in-hospital care must be considered.

More often than not delays for resuscitation and preparation are beneficial, but delays should be permitted only to improve the patient's condition. Occasionally, for instance when there is massive continuing haemorrhage, as in some ruptured spleens and ruptured ectopic pregnancies when transfusion cannot keep pace with loss, and even if the blood pressure is raised it may only increase the loss still further, it may be better to stop the bleeding surgically and transfuse afterwards.

The emergency treatment of obstruction of the upper airway

Accidental total obstruction of the upper air passages will lead first to hypoxia, then to respiratory arrest due to depression of the respiratory centre and finally to cardiac arrest and irreversible brain damage. The time available for action after sudden total respiratory obstruction to inevitable death is possibly about 8 min; this is fortunately rather longer than after primary cardiac arrest and instantaneous cessation of the circulation, when it is probably about 4 min. Immediate action is required whether the patient is in an everyday environment away from the hospital or in the hospital itself.

Partial obstruction is recognised by cyanosis, tachycardia (until hypoxia causes bradycardia), laryngeal tug, heaving respiration with indrawing of the intercostal, supraclavicular and suprasternal spaces. Characteristically, the abdomen and chest move up and down alternately in a 'see-saw' movement.[1]

Obstruction from pressure on the outside of the upper airway is comparatively infrequent. In the acute situation outside the hospital, constriction due to the rope of suicidal hanging may be encountered, and in the hospital, haematoma in a recent thyroidectomy wound is an example. In either case, the treatment is to remove the cause — by removing the ligature or opening and evacuating the wound. The old first aid instruction to 'loosen the clothing at the neck' has less application in these days of soft collars.

---

[1] The nursing aphorism still holds; that 'noisy breathing is obstructed, and obstructed breathing is noisy' except with total obstruction.

Obstruction from the walls of the airway is most often due to the jaw and tongue falling back and obstructing the laryngopharynx in the unconscious patient. Extension of the head and pushing the jaw forward are manoeuvres carried out constantly in the daily practice of the anaesthetist (Chapter 6, Fig. 6.1). Failure to wipe out debris from the throat and to perform this simple manoeuvre has frequently caused the death of unconscious accident victims. The oropharyngeal airway is as useful in the first aid situation as it is in the operating theatre. Once the airway is assured, the spontaneously breathing patient should be turned on his side into the safe position. Tracheal intubation is increasingly taught to paramedical ambulance personnel as an advanced first aid manoeuvre for securing the airway of unconscious patients for transportation and to facilitate IPPV.

Maxillofacial trauma may cause partial obstruction which can be relieved by positioning the head and neck or tracheal intubation, but occasionally complete obstruction occurs which can be relieved only by tracheotomy or cricothyrotomy (the opening of the larynx below the cords through the cricothyroid membrane — see below).

Obstruction in the lumen of the upper air passages is frequently from secretions or the debris of trauma (blood, broken teeth,) which can be removed by wiping out or sucking out the mouth. A much more dangerous situation can be caused by a foreign body obstructing the glottis.

Many restaurants in the USA display posters illustrating the action which should be taken if a diner gets a piece of food firmly lodged in the glottis. The patient should be first laid on his side (or in the case of a child, held head down) and struck between the shoulder blades in the hope of dislodging the bolus (this manoeuvre should not be undertaken with the patient sitting up as the obstruction may pass into the lower respiratory tract under gravity). If this fails, the

Heimlich manoeuvre should be tried — if the patient is still conscious the operator stands behind the casualty with his arms round his body and the hands clasped over the epigastrium. A sharp pull upwards and backward may raise the intrathoracic pressure to such an extent that the bolus is forced out of the glottis like a cork from a bottle. If the patient is unconscious, the manoeuvre can be performed frcm the front by similar sharp pressure in the epigastrium with the patient supine. If the Heimlich manoeuvre fails the only recourse is cricothyrotomy.

Cricothyrotomy. Cricothyrotomy will by-pass an obstruction at or above the vocal cords. Total obstruction has occasionally been described when a dental sponge or dam has lodged in the back of the pharynx after its safety tape has snapped — such blood soaked and slimy objects are unlikely to be expelled by the Heimlich manoeuvre and cricothyrotomy is immediately necessary. Cricothyrotomy may also be indicated when total obstruction results from rapid oedema of the glottis (as in an acute anaphylatic reaction to a drug) from maxillofacial trauma or very severe laryngeal spasm. Fortunately, spasm can usually be overcome by ensuring that the upper airway is clear and applying 100% oxygen under pressure. Maxillofacial trauma and glottic oedema generally give rise to partial obstruction; this is potentially dangerous but not immediately life threatening and can be relieved by tracheostomy.

The cricothyroid membrane can be felt in the depression between the prominence of the thyroid cartilage (the Adam's apple) and the ring of the cricoid cartilage. It is superficial. In an emergency, away from the hospital, a penknife (held about 1.5 cm from the tip to avoid it passing through the larynx) can be used to make an opening into the larynx of the unconcious but unanaesthetised patient and any suitable tubular object can be inserted (e.g. one of the cricothyrotomy trocar and cannula devices from the paramedic's kit, 5 cm of stethoscope tubing, the barrel of a ball point pen with the refill removed, etc.)[2].

In a hospital where large bore needles or intravenous cannulae are readily available, several can be inserted. If oxygen is applied to such a needle a second needle must be in place to act as a safety valve to avoid build up in pressure and possible rupture of the lung.

Tracheostomy may be indicated for partial obstruction of the upper airway (maxillofacial injuries, oedema of the glottis, laryngopharyngeal tumours, foreign bodies, etc.), to provide access for the removal of secretions in the lower respiratory tract, or to facilitate prolonged IPPV in the intensive care unit. Obviously, it will be mandatory if the obstruction lies in the larynx below the cricoid cartilage and thus below the site for cricothyrotomy.

Tracheostomy is a more complicated surgical procedure than cricothyrotomy because of various structures related to the trachea including the thyroid isthmus. It is obviously a better procedure if the lower respiratory tract has to be intubated for a prolonged period. In partial obstruction the patient is likely to be conscious and will require general or local anaesthesia.

Local anaesthesia can be used for tracheostomy and is particularly indicated if it is not possible to pass a tracheal tube, however small in diameter, through the mouth or nose before the operation of tracheostomy is undertaken. Subcutaneous infiltration in the line of the incision is followed by deeper injection into tissues of the midline, thus producing

---

[2] The barrel of a plastic syringe inserted by a Royal Army Medical Corps Sergeant saved the life of a soldier shot in the neck in the Northern Ireland emergency. Over 80 cricothyrotomies were performed by paramedical personnel for maxillofacial injuries in Vietnam. An American lady physician trapped in an automobile crash on an isolated road in California attempted to open her own cricothyroid membrane with a pocket knife but sadly failed to do so.

a painless track from skin to trachea. The anaesthetist should assist by monitoring the patient's condition and giving encouragement and oxygen. Sedation may be required through a secure intravenous needle using a benzodiazepine such as midazolam, but great care should be taken to avoid the respiratory depressant effects of the drugs.

General anaesthesia is commonly preferred for tracheostomy but can be dangerous if it is not possible to intubate the patient's trachea beforehand. Many deaths have occurred in the past at the moment of insertion of the tracheostomy tube. A venous cannula is inserted and sedation which does not depress respiration (diazepam 0.5 mg–5.0 mg or midazolam 0.25 mg–2.5 mg) is given cautiously. If there is an obstruction, spontaneous respiration should be maintained until it is certain that the obstruction can be removed or bypassed. The technique of gaseous induction of anaesthesia can be used after preoxygenation; the concentration of halothane or enflurane are gradually increased to 3–5%, so that laryngoscopy can be tolerated. If there is an obstruction, the anaesthetist may be able to see an obstructing foreign body and remove it with Magill's forceps. If he cannot remove the foreign body, or the obstruction is in the wall of the airway, and he can see his way to placing a tracheal tube under direct vision, he should do so, preferably after spraying local anaesthetic onto the larynx and vocal cords. Once the tube is securely placed in the trachea, adequate oxygenation should be possible and tracheostomy can be undertaken relatively leisurely. The anaesthetist's tracheal tube should be partially withdrawn and kept with its tip just below the vocal cords until it is certain that the tracheostomy tube is in the trachea and adequate respiration can take place through it. Such a precaution is necessary as the surgeon may have difficulty and miss the trachea altogether when inserting a tracheostomy tube.

Foreign bodies in the lower respiratory tract. Unrelieved

obstruction of the trachea by an inhaled foreign body is usually fatal, but fortunately, because of the narrow passage between the cords, inhaled solid foreign bodies such as a nut or tooth are small enough also to pass down into one or other bronchus — usually the right because of the straighter anatomical configuration. Anaesthesia for the removal of foreign bodies below the cords can prove difficult and potentially dangerous, particularly as the patient is often a child with a narrow airway. The principles of anaesthetic management described above for tracheostomy apply — intravenous access, adequate monitoring and avoidance of paralysis or controlled ventilaton which may force the foreign body further down the respiratory tract. Deep anaesthesia is required to overcome the sensitive tracheal and bronchial reflexes. A rigid bronchoscope is used with a side channel through which oxygen and anaesthetic mixture may be added.

Mediastinal shift

The mediastinum can be deflected and cause respiratory embarrassment and severe shock if air or blood accumulates in the hemithorax under tension. The first aid treatment is to insert a chest drain to empty the hemithorax. It will then be safer to anaesthetise the patient and not risk increasing the mediastinal shift from the leak of gases used under pressure to ventilate the patient.

Hypovolaemia

The administration of anaesthesia to the hypovolaemic patient is risky. The unanaesthetised patient can compensate to a remarkable degree for loss of blood volume by sympatheticoadrenal discharge causing vasoconstriction. A fit young man can lose up to 30% of his blood volume without a fall in blood pressure — indeed, his blood pressure may actually rise due to over compensation. As soon as he is anaesthetised these compensatory vasoconstrictive powers are suppressed, the vascular bed dilates, the blood pressure will plummet, profound hypotension will ensue, the coronary circulation will be markedly reduced and the patient may die.

Blood volume may be lost because of loss of electrolyes (into the gut in intestinal obstruction for example), or of plasma (as in cases of second degree burns where large areas of body surface are affected) or of whole blood. Electrolyte losses and plasma (colloid) losses must be replaced with appropriate fluids. Discussion in this chapter will be devoted primarily to consideration of whole blood loss (haemorrhage).

Haemorrhage

Haemorrhage can be 'revealed' or 'concealed' or both.

Revealed haemorrhage is assessed by examination of body surface wounds and observation of blood losses from haemoptysis, melaena or haematemesis (though in the case of loss into the stomach or gut, the amount voided may be only a small fraction of the total loss into the gastrointestinal system).

Concealed haemorrhage into a body cavity such as the peritoneum (ruptured ectopic pregnancy, rupture of the spleen), the retroperitoneal space (kidney) or the pleural space (haemothorax), or loss into closed fracture sites is difficult to estimate and may escape notice until cardiovascular collapse occurs.

Multiple trauma

The management of the multiple trauma patient highlights many of the problems of blood volume replacement.

Immediate treatment is devoted to eliminating any potential threat to life (respiratory obstruction, pneumothorax and haemorrhage). Oxygen should be administered, the airway of the unconscious patient should be secured by intubation (great care being taken if there is any possibility of injury to the cervical spine) and ventilation controlled, if this is threatened.

Blood volume replacement. Obvious major bleeding points should be controlled by compression. At least two intravenous cannulae should be inserted percutaneously or by cut-down. A specimen of blood should be taken and sent for grouping and crossmatch at the same time. If the patient is exsanguinated and pulseless, it is best to start the infusion with a litre of normal saline or Hartmann's Ringer lactate solution to avoid intravascular coagulation due to sludging. Otherwise, colloid should be used — human albumen solution (HAS), gelatin solution (Haemaccel®), dextran 70 in 0.9% saline or hetastarch (Hespan®). Hetastarch is probably the best choice as an artificial plasma expander, as its high molecular weight ensures it will stay in circulation for an appreciable length of time; it also triggers few anaphylactic reactions and does not alter blood coagulability. Blood is substituted as soon as available but the essential need is for volume replacement not haemoglobin — indeed the 'ideal' haemoglobin for oxygen availability to the tissues is nearer 30% than the 'normal' 45% because reduced viscosity increases the rate of perfusion.

Analgesia, best titrated intravenously, should be given to the conscious patient, due regard being paid to avoiding compromising respiration or consciousness. Intravenous morphia is efficacious.

Monitoring and recording should be started at once and include frequent assessment of level of consciousness and responsiveness, pupil size and reaction, pulse rate, arterial blood pressure, electrocardiogram and urinary output from an indwelling catheter. A central venous line should be inserted as soon as is practicable (see below).

Assessment of loss of blood volume is the next step when

immediate danger to life has been eliminated and rapid infusion of colloid solution has been initiated. Blood loss in multiple trauma cases is often underestimated; by the time the patient has reached the Accident and Emergency Department, much blood may have been left on the ground and soaked up in the clothing and stretcher coverings whilst current bleeding is greatly reduced by hypotension. A method of estimating 'revealed' haemorrhage is to make an estimate from examination of the open wounds — tissue damage equivalent in volume to the clenched adult fist represents a loss of 500 ml and skin loss equivalent to the size of the patient's hand represents a loss of 10% of blood volume (500 ml for the adult).

Concealed haemorrhage is more difficult to assess and losses into closed fracture sites can be very large (for example, for fractures in the adult, pelvis 1000–2000 ml, femoral shaft 1000 ml, tibia 500 ml, bones of the upper limb 200–300 ml, each fractured rib 120 ml). Several litres can be lost into the abdomen (either into the peritoneal cavity itself or the retroperitoneal space), and be difficult to detect — peritoneal lavage and abdominal distension are unreliable signs. Rib fractures overlying viscera (spleen, liver, kidneys) lead to suspicion of possible rupture of the organs. Widening of the mediastinum may indicate a haematoma or a ruptured aorta, and a displacement of the mediastinum a haemothorax. Shadows in the lung fields may indicate haemothorax or lung contusion but the absence of radiological signs does not exclude them.

Central venous pressure (CVP) is measured either by a simple saline manometer or electronically by recording the pressure of the tip of a long catheter placed in a great vein near the heart. This represents the pressure in the right atrium and thus the ventricular end diastolic pressure (VEDP). The absolute value of this measurement (2–12 cm H_2O) is less important than its response to the challenge of fluid infusion. If the patient is normovolaemic, it will rise some 2–3 cm H_2O, (for example, from 10 cm H_2O–12.5 cm H_2O) in response to a rapid 'challenge' of fluid of approximately 2 ml/kg and then drop back to its original value over 4–5 min. If the patient is hypervolaemic (overtransfused) the pressure will rise 2 or 3 cm H_2O and stay at that level. If the patient is still hypovolaemic (i.e. replacement of blood loss is inadequate) the initial value is low (say 0 to 1 cm H_2O) and it will rise little, if at all, in response to the challenge. A persistently low CVP in response to apparently adequate replacement of estimated revealed haemorrhage should lead to suspicion that there is some concealed source of haemorrhage. A high CVP amid a low arterial blood pressure in response to obviously adequate volume replacement indicates that the heart is failing and requires pharmacological support, or possibly that there is cardiac tamponade.

Urinary output is a useful indicator of adequate cardiac output (and thus of adequate blood replacement) provided the kidneys have not been damaged by prolonged hypotension. This can be suspected if there is a high CVP in response to adequate replacement but urinary output remains low (less than 0.5 ml per kg body weight per hour).

Complications of massive blood transfusion. The transfusion of cold stored blood brings the potential complications of hypothermia and reduced cardiac output. Blood which is to be given rapidly should be warmed to 37°C by passing it through a coil immersed in a water bath. Warming the blood will also speed up the intravascular buffering process counteracting the acidity of stored blood, promote the release of ionised calcium removed by the chemical anticoagulant and restore potassium to the cells from the plasma. Stored blood also contains microaggregates of platelets and other cellular debris which should be filtered out as they may cause pulmonary damage. The processes for infection screening in the United Kingdom are excellent, but elsewhere the possibilities of hepatitis B, HIV (AIDS), viral infections and malaria, etc., must be borne in mind. Stored blood near its expiring date will be deficient in platelets and clotting factors — supplementation with fresh blood or special blood products may be required.

Losses of colloid from burns and crystalloid from intestinal obstruction, etc. must be estimated and replaced with the appropriate fluid. The loss of colloid from burns will be continuous over the first 36 h. Formulae are used to estimate losses from deep burn surfaces (for example 3 × percentage of body surface area of burns × body weight in the first 36 hours — half to be replaced in the first 12 h, one third in the second 12 h and one sixth in the third 12 h). An adult patient who is clinically dehydrated (thirst, furred tongue, inelastic tissues, etc.), is probably deficient in at least 3000 ml of crystalloid (about 4% of body weight).

Anaesthesia and hypovolaemia. It is usually possible to gain on blood loss and improve the patient's condition, but in some cases of internal arterial blood loss (aortic aneurysms, ruptured ectopic pregnancy, ruptured spleens. etc.) it is not possible and anaesthesia must be given in the face of hypovolaemic shock. Great care and careful titration of dosage is necessary as the lowered volume enhances the action of intravenous agents. Drugs which tend to raise or preserve cardiac output and blood pressure (ketamine, etomidate, pancuronium, etc.) should be used.

Emergencies in abdominal surgery

The problem of the full stomach is one that overshadows all emergency anaesthetics because gastric stasis always accompanies the physical and mental stress of a bodily emergency; when the surgical condition is abdominal the dangers are compounded. The danger is that regurgitated stomach contents aspirated into the lungs causes considerable pulmonary damage related to the quantity and acidity of the aspirate (Mendelson's syndrome). We are concerned in this chapter with prevention of this dire complication. Its treatment will be considered in Chapter 13.

If an individual is fit and starved of solid food for 6 h and fluids for 2 h, his stomach will be empty except for about 20 ml of residue. But many conditions, including trauma and late pregnancy, and labour (see Chapter 10), will delay emptying. A child who falls from a tree shortly after a meal and fractures his arm may retain his food in his stomach for many hours undigested and identifiable. In intestinal obstruction, the stomach will even fill in a retrograde fashion from the small intestine. It is safest to assume that every patient presenting for an emergency anaesthetic has a full stomach and to act accordingly.

A number of precautions can be taken:-

1. A nasogastric tube (16 gauge for the adult) can be inserted. It is obviously fanciful to believe that fish and chips can be removed through a tube small enough to be passed through the nose, but the nasogastric tube is useful in releasing fluid or gas. If left in place, it may make the lower oesophageal sphincter incompetent and increase the risk of aspiration. Passage of a large bore orogastric tube is likely to be tolerated only by patients who are inebriated or unconscious.

2. Metoclopramide (10 mg intramuscularly or intravenously) increases gastric motility and enhances lower oesophageal sphincter tone, but its effectiveness is reduced by prior atropine administration. Dysrhythmias may occur if the intravenous injection is too rapid.

3. The secretion of acid in gastric juice can be reduced by H_2 histamine receptor blockers. The worst damage to lung tissue comes from inhalation of gastric contents with pH less than 2.5. The most satisfactory drug is ranitidine

150 mg intramuscularly or by mouth at least two hours before operation. Cimetidine 300 mg (slowly intravenously, intramuscularly or by mouth), which is more rapid in onset but shorter acting, can also be used but it is less effective. These reduce the volume and acidity of gastric juice secreted after they have been administered but obviously will have no effect on the gastric acid already present.

4. An antacid can be given but should be chosen with care. Magnesium trisilicate has been traditionally used, but it mixes poorly with the stomach juices, causes lung damage itself if aspirated, and though a good buffer its effectiveness deteriorates with storage. It is being superseded by sodium citrate (20–30 ml of 0.3 molar solution flavoured with peppermint and saccharine). Sodium citrate acts rapidly but transiently, it is relatively benign if aspirated into the lungs and is best given within 20 minutes of induction of anaesthesia. 20 ml of sodium bicarbonate 8.4% (a solution readily available because it is used for cardiac resuscitation) is also effective.

The prevention of regurgitation and aspiration during anaesthesia. There are three methods of dealing with the problem.

1. *Inhalation induction* with the head tilted down and the patient on his side. This is an old fashioned but well tried method which can still be useful, especially if the patient is in a moribund condition. It was used extensively before the introduction of muscle relaxants increased the danger from passive regurgitation. The patient quite often vomits actively but does so at a stage when the protective reflexes of the larynx are still present.

2. *Awake intubation under local anaesthesia.* This was at one time much favoured in the United States but can be unpleasant for the patient if not carried out with expertise.

3. *Rapid sequence induction,* the method almost universally practised in the United Kingdom — preoxygenation,

intravenous induction, relaxation with suxamethonium, intubation. Rapid sequence induction is now invariably (and rightly) accompanied by cricothyroid pressure (Sellick's manoeuvre — described in 1961) to occlude the oesophagus.

Cricothyroid pressure (Sellick's manoeuvre). The cricoid is the only laryngeal cartilage which completely encircles the larynx. It is triangular in cross-section with a flat posterior surface. Pressure directly backwards on the cricoid directed towards the cervical vertebrae will therefore occlude the oesophagus and prevent fluid from passing into the pharynx, and thus being aspirated into the larynx. Although the manoeuvre appears simple, it demands accurate and practised positioning of the assistant's hands, which may obstruct the laryngoscope, distort the normal anatomy of the larynx or fail to occlude the oesophagus. If the patient vomits actively (wholly different from passive insiduous regurgitation) the cricoid pressure must be released or the oesophagus might be ruptured. A patient who can vomit between the administration of the induction agent and the suxamethonium usually retains enough reflex activity to guard his own airway, and will be safe providing an effective suction apparatus can clear the vomitus from the pharynx before he takes his next, and potentially last, breath.

Pre-oxygenation is essential before rapid sequence induction of anaesthesia. It serves three purposes:-

1. Nitrogen is eliminated, thus increasing the reserves of oxygen and permitting a longer period of apnoea.
2. The anaesthetist need not hand-ventilate the patient with a mask after neuromuscular block has been produced. There is therefore less delay before tracheal intubation, and oxygen is not forced into the stomach thus increasing both the intra-gastric pressure and the risk of regurgitation.
3. In the longer term, nitrogen in distended bowel may be reduced so decreasing abdominal pressure.

Rapid sequence induction is of fundamental importance to modern anaesthetic practice, the details are as follows:-
1. *Equipment* (tested and in working order):-
   Tilting trolley or operating table which can be operated with one hand.
   Suction apparatus
   Two laryngoscopes
   Two cuffed tracheal tubes, introducers and connectors
   Anaesthetic apparatus
   Oxygen supply, face mask and means of giving oxygen under pressure.
   ECG. Heart rate and blood pressure monitors.
2. *Personnel*
   Anaesthetist
   Anaesthetic assistant trained in the use of all apparatus and cricoid pressure.
   Surgeon, scrubbed and ready
   Ward nurse
3. *Posture*.
   Supine, (the patient must never be induced in the lithotomy position — this raises intragastric pressure (as do obesity, heavy bedclothes on the abdomen, or gravid uterus which also distorts the gastric anatomy).
4. *Preoxygenation*
   10 l/min for 3 min or 5 maximum voluntary breaths
5. *Induction*
   Intravenous infusion running freely
   Pretreatment with tubocurarine 3 mg or gallamine 20 mg
   Cricoid pressure after warning patient
   Thiopentone followed by suxamethonium[3]
   Continued cricoid pressure.

---

[3] Suxamethonium increases intragastric pressure during depolarisation by as much as 120 cm H_2O but recent work shows that it also contracts the cardiac sphincter.

6. *Intubation*
   Continued cricoid pressure
   Laryngoscopy
   Intubation with tube on semi-rigid introducer
   Cuff inflated by assistant to airtight seal
   Assistant releases cricoid pressure when told to do so
   Position of tube checked for possible bronchial intubation
   and repositioned if necessary.
   Tube secured
7. *Maintenance of anaesthesia*
   Long acting competitive blocking agents when suxame-
   thonium wears off
   Controlled ventilation with O_2: N_2O and minimal volatile
   agent
8. *Emergence and extubation*
   Reversal of muscle relaxant with atropine and prostigmine.
   Head down on left side
   Suction and oxygen ready to hand
   (regurgitation is still possible)
   Extubate when able to cough

Appendicectomy is probably the commonest abdominal
emergency. Many patients will have vomited and probably
emptied their stomachs but the rapid induction sequence
should be followed meticulously. The operation should not
be undertaken lightly as it may unexpectedly become a major
procedure; beware especially of patients with a long history
of symptoms before coming to surgery — dehydration,
metabolic acidosis, and hypokalaemia may all have developed
insiduously and unnoticed, and should be corrected
preoperatively.

Intestinal obstruction is a serious condition and particularly
so in the elderly, who may have additional cardiopulmonary
problems. Hydrochloric acid, fluid and potassium have all
been lost. The patient may be hypovolaemic, dehydrated,
oliguric, hypokalaemic, and have a metabolic acidosis. These

must be corrected before induction of anaesthesia because of the enhanced problems of hypotension, renal failure, dysrhythmias and inability to withstand further fluid loss or myocardial depression.

Monitoring is important. A central venous pressure line and an indwelling urinary catheter should be inserted and measurements from these, together with aspiration from a nasogastric tube, will provide a reasonable indication of the state of hydration. Intravenous fluids should be infused until at least 0.5 ml/kg of urine/hour is produced and the CVP should reach 3–5 cm H_2O. The blood pressure and heart rate should be within the patient's normal limits before the induction of anaesthesia. The tilt test or sit-up test are useful for assessing the adequacy of fluid replacement. There should be no change in systemic blood pressure when the patient is moved from the horizontal to the sitting position or tilted head down.

Intestinal obstruction usually produces grossly distended bowel. Although the surgeon may decompress the bowel and reduce its bulk, it may still be difficult to pack back into the abdomen at the end of the operation. Good muscle relaxation is, therefore, required just when the anaesthetist is wanting to reverse the neuromuscular block and restore spontaneous ventilation. The surgeon may unwittingly improve relaxation by instilling large amounts of aminoglycoside antibiotics (which potentiate competitive neuromuscular block) into the peritoneal cavity.

Reversal of neuromuscular blockade is usually achieved with a mixture of atropine and neostigmine. It is suggested that anticholinesterase drugs, by increasing gut motility, may put undue stress on tenuous suture lines of bowel anastomoses and make the anastomosis leak; it is sometimes possible by judicious use of the newer neuromuscular blockers (atracurium and vecuronium) to avoid having to use neostigmine.

Peripheral vascular emergencies

Leaking aortic aneurysms are often fatal however treated. The anaesthetist may contribute to the mortality by failure to plan properly. If the aorta leaks blood into the peritoneal cavity the abdomen will eventually become tense. The intra-abdominal pressure will equal the already reduced aortic pressure and loss of blood will then cease — until the anaesthetist relaxes the tight abdominal muscles and allows the patient to bleed through the aorta again.

The patient should first be positioned on the operating table. Intravascular monitoring established (CVP and arterial lines inserted under local anaesthesia) and the skin prepared and the operation site draped before anaesthesia is induced.

Rapid sequence intubation is employed (using ketamine or etomidate rather than thiopentone to avoid drugs which may precipitate hypotension). Once the airway is secured by intubation, and with a brisk infusion of blood running, the surgeon should swiftly open the abdomen, grasp the aorta above the leak and apply a cross-clamp. The anaesthetist can then hope to begin to restore the blood volume by transfusion.

The high risk of oligaemic renal failure can be reduced by as rapid restoration of circulating blood volume as possible, and osmotic diuretics such as mannitol 125–250 ml or frusemide 20–40 mg may be given intravenously to promote a diuresis.

Peripheral vascular disease may present as an emergency from acute occlusion of the blood supply to the lower limbs by an embolised clot or fragment of atheroma. The patient may also have recently had an operation on the more proximal blood vessels and be a diabetic or a chronic bronchitic, or be in atrial fibrillation (see Chapter 12).

Surgical emergencies from peripheral vascular disease can often be managed under regional anaesthesia and sedation. Concurrent use of anticoagulants prohibits epidural blockade.

Hypotension must be avoided in patients who already have a compromised blood supply.

Transplantation surgery. Modern techniques of organ preservation have reduced the previous urgency of transplantation. It must be remembered that many recipients are blissfully unaware that a compatible organ is soon to be available while they continue their daily life. All recipients not already in hospital should therefore be regarded as having a 'full stomach'.

The anaesthetist avoids placing intravenous or intra-arterial cannula at sites which may be needed for arteriovenous shunts. Internal jugular venous lines are preferred. Immuno-suppressive drugs may be required and immaculate asepsis should be practised.

Gynaecological emergencies

Ectopic pregnancies are usually diagnosed earlier than they used to be because the patients undergo laparoscopy to confirm or exclude the diagnosis. Massive bleeding and aspiration of stomach contents is still a possibility and patients must be managed with care along the lines already described.

Evacuation of the retained products of conception is a common procedure which is not always treated with the respect it deserves. These patients are apt to be relegated to the end of a full day's operating list and allocated to the least experienced surgeon and anaesthetist. Some patients will bleed to the point of needing transfusion; regurgitation of acid gastric secretions is always a possibility.

Obstetric emergencies

This subject has already been considered in Chapter 10. All general anaesthetics for obstetrics must be regarded as emergencies and conducted with particular attention to all the points detailed earlier in the chapter for the management of anaesthesia for patients with a full stomach. General anaesthesia has the advantage over regional of being swift and certain, but an incidence of maternal awareness (as high as 17.5% in some series) has been reported because of the desire of anaesthetists to use as little volatile agent as possible in order not to compromise the fetus.

Regional anaesthesia is contraindicated in the presence of third trimester bleeding because of the risk of producing irreversible hypotension, but apart from this, it is increasingly chosen for emergency obstetrics. The mother remains awake and aware for the delivery: a circumstance which is believed to be helpful in the maternal-child bonding process. Spinal block is also increasingly commonly used, but has the disadvantages of a single-shot technique and is applicable only if there is no hypovolaemia, as the sympathetic block which it produces causes hypotension.

Epidural blockade established through an indwelling catheter, is adjustable (unlike a spinal block). It can be extended if it proves inadequate, and can be prolonged for postoperative pain relief.

Surgical emergencies in the neonate

There is no place for unpractised anaesthetists or surgeons in the surgery for neonates (see Chapter 10). Whenever feasible, the infant should be transported to the nearest neonatal centre, while kept warm, oxygenated and hydrated.

Orthopaedic emergencies

Fractures are common, especially amongst the elderly and infirm. A fracture at some sites may compromise local blood supply and need immediate reduction to prevent permanent ischaemic damage. Most fractures can be stabilised and

immobilised without anaesthesia until preoperative preparation is complete. Upper limb fractures can frequently and
advantageously be treated by local anaesthetic methods
(Chapter 9).

Fractured hips typically occur in frail, elderly women.
When they present for surgery they are hypovolaemic,
anaemic and ill prepared with multiple inadequately treated
medical conditions. There may be conflict between
attempting to improve the general medical condition of the
patient while allowing the risks of pulmonary problems,
embolism of fat or clot, and the threat to skin under pressure,
to be magnified by the delay. Early ambulation is desirable,
hence early operation is required. The choice of anaesthetic
technique is controversial. Ironically, whatever technique is
chosen — anaesthetic, spinal or epidural block, the mortality
at three months remains around 30%. Reduction in arterial
carbon dioxide tension brought about by IPPV may impair
cerebral perfusion.

Neurosurgery

Intracranial disasters — subdural or subarachnoid haemorrhage, cerebral abscess or intracranial tumours all present as
emergencies when the intracranial pressure is dangerously
raised. Decompression by trephining burr holes is indicated
followed by removal of the clot or abscess, for which a flap
of bone and scalp may have to be moved. This may be
undertaken under local anaesthesia. If general anaesthesia is
required, intracranial pressure can be reduced by hyperventilation, increased oxygenation, posture, diuretics, and
systemic steroids, and if necessary by spinal drainage of CSF.
It is best to avoid volatile halogenated anaesthetic agents as
they may raise intracranial pressure and produce prolonged
unconsciousness. Central nervous system depressant drugs
may cloud the patient's consciousness, and only short acting

intravenous agents should be used. Thiopentone and fentanyl (with nitrous oxide and neuromuscular block) usually ensure rapid return of consciousness — assuming that the brain has not been irretrievably damaged.

Fracture dislocation of the neck may result from the whiplash injury of a motor car accident. Movement of the neck may cause permanent high spinal damage. Neck movement should be minimised by skull traction attached to a weight. Neurological signs should be checked before and after anaesthesia. If the neurological and recorded signs and symptoms are worsened by trivial movement before anaesthesia has been induced, tracheostomy is necessary under local anaesthesia if general anaesthesia is required for other surgical problems.

Emergencies in thoracic surgery

An empyaema connected to the bronchial tree is traditionally at first dealt with by rib resection and drainage under intercostal block with the patient sitting upright. The patient retains his cough reflex and cross aspiration into the other lung is prevented.

The closure of a bronchopleural fistula presents a particular anaesthetic problem in that IPPV may produce a tension pneumothorax due to gases escaping through the fistula. Either a cuffed bronchial tube must be introduced into the opposite main bronchus under direct vision or, better, prior insertion of an underwater sealed drainage tube into the affected side will prevent a tension pneumothorax from being formed the enable IPPV to be used from the start.

Ear, nose and throat emergencies

Bleeding from the tonsillar fossa occurs postoperatively from time to time even after surgery by the most careful surgeon.

The condition is life threatening because of the haemorrhage itself, much of which may be concealed by swallowing[4], and because of the possibility of respiratory obstruction, from either direct aspiration or regurgitated stomach contents with the additional possibility of acid damage.

The general principles of anaesthetising any patient apply. Prior transfusion is mandatory even though the surgeon may understandably be anxious to remedy the problem. Some anaesthetists prefer to carry out inhalation induction before intubation, with the patient in the lateral position, especially with small children. Others opt for the rapid sequence induction technique with the patient head down and turned to the left and cricoid pressure applied.

Oral surgery

Trismus. Infection in the mouth can cause trismus. Spontaneous respiration with an inhalational induction should always be employed in the presence of trismus unless there is evidence of glottic oedema as well, when a nasotracheal tube should be passed under local anaesthesia — not a technique for the inexperienced anaesthetist.

Fractured jaw. If the jaws are to be wired together to stabilise the fractures, or if there is persistent intraoral bleeding, the nasotracheal tube should be left in place until the patient is sufficiently awake and the protective laryngopharyngeal reflexes return. The patient can then be asked to remove his own endotracheal tube. Wire cutters should

[4] One of the authors recalls the case of a fit sailor in a military hospital in the 1950's who bled to death during the night after a tonsillectomy when a ligature slipped. There was very little blood on the victim's pillow.

always be at hand in case of emergency. It is better to save life even if it means incurring the displeasure of the surgeon.[5].

---

[5] One of the authors had his life put at risk by a patient who gagged in the process of extubating himself after his jaws had been wired together for a fractured mandible, and then went into laryngospasm as the tube passed out of the cords. The patient, who was sitting up in bed at the time and was previously alert and cooperative, grabbed the author's throat with both hands and squeezed. Thus, the patient and the anaesthetist rapidly became hypoxic together. The author's arms were not long enough to reach the patient's face or tube, as he was held at a long arms' length by the patient. Another anaesthetist chanced to enter the room, appraised the situation, decided on his priorities, and deftly reinserted the patient's nasotracheal tube. The patient's hypoxic grasp was relieved and all could breath again. Be warned, always stand behind the head of a patient whom you can not control!

12

Disease and anaesthesia

'Common sense is the basis of good anaesthesia — but then, so is it the foundation of all medicine'.

Anaesthesia for Medical Students. First edition, 1949.

Many diseases, and the drugs used to treat them, affect the conduct of anaesthesia, and so the differences in technique and management which they demand must be taken into account. This chapter will discuss some of these problems, whether real or anticipated. It is very important that all those associated with prescription for surgical patients, especially house surgeons, should be aware of the difficulties.

Conditions affecting the central nervous system

Epilepsy. Anticonvulsant drugs such as phenytoin and carbamazepine may induce hepatic metabolic enzymes and enhance breakdown of some drugs, producing shortened and reduced actions. Gingival hyperplasia is common in patients chronically treated with phenytoin; gums may bleed easily and teeth are more readily loosened. The anaesthetist must be aware of these problems but anticonvulsants should not be discontinued before anaesthesia. The 'stress' of hospitalization and the mistaken omission of the usual dose of anticonvulsant drug preoperatively increase risk of epileptic

183

convulsion. Enflurane, methohexitone, ketamine and over-doses of local anaesthetics are all potentially convulsive and best used with caution in epileptic patients. Diazepam and thiopentone are useful anticonvulsants, and being commonly used in anaesthesia, epileptic convulsions are rarely seen in the perioperative period.

Down's syndrome is associated with a large tongue, a narrow larynx and instability of the cervical spine, so that intubation and airway management may be difficult and even dangerous. Preoperative cervical X-rays are necessary to assess the spine.

Mental subnormality may make cooperation unlikely. Time spent gaining the confidence of the patient and obtaining the help from whomsoever accompanies him is well spent. An electrocardiogram may demonstrate associated cardiac conduction defects. Intramuscular ketamine may be the best way to manage the induction of an uncooperative subnormal patient.

Deafness and/or blindness. Co-operation during procedures under local anaesthesia may be difficult for those suffering from deafness and/or blindness. All staff must be made aware of the patient's disability. Sympathetic recovery staff should help the patient to regain his orientation as consciousness returns.

Drug addicted patients can be manipulative and may seek to obtain additional doses of addictive drugs while in hospital. They should be given their usual dosage plus whatever other analgesic or sedative regimen is habitually used for ordinary patients. There is a risk of hepatitis B and HIV infection from the use of unsterilised needles, and 'main-line' addicts may have poor veins.

Depression. Monoamine oxidase inhibitor therapy is fortunately less favoured by psychiatrists than it was in the past. These drugs should be discontinued three weeks preoperatively because of the danger of inducing coma and respiratory

depression if opioids are administered and of hypertension
with indirectly acting sympathomimetic pressor drugs, such
as methoxamine, phenylephrine, etc. Other antidepressants
(but not tricyclics which are also liable to cause cardiac irregularities and hypertension) should be substituted. Psychiatrists are sometimes loath to alter a combination that has
proved effective. Pancuronium, halothane or ephedrine and
other indirectly acting pressor agents should be avoided, as
these enhance the uptake of catecholamines released from
sympathetic nerve endings and may produce intractable
cardiac dysrhythmias. Other means of controlling postoperative pain should be employed, including local anaesthesia
(without adrenaline).

Raised intracranial pressure and depressed consiousness. Long
acting central nervous system depressant drugs should be
avoided. Atropine alone should be used for premedication.
The anaesthetist must aim to have the patient as awake at the
end of procedure as before induction. Hyperventilation
reduces arterial carbon dioxide and thus intracranial pressure.
'Smooth' anaesthesia, by eliminating coughing, bucking, and
straining, decreases the risk of increasing intracranial pressure
further.

Conditions affecting the spinal cord and the peripheral nervous system

*Paraplegia, hemiplegia, prolonged immobilisation and polio-
myelitis.* Hyperkalaemia severe enough to cause dysrhythmias
and even cardiac arrest may follow the use of suxamethonium
because of the release of potassium due to pathological alterations in muscle metabolism. Pretreatment with a small dose
of non-depolarizer (e.g. tubocurarine) is said to reduce the
problem, but it is better to avoid use of suxamethonium
altogether.

Extra care is necessary in positioning these patients because lack of the ability to appreciate pain may allow undue pressure to be tolerated.

Multiple sclerosis. The variable nature of this disease with its remissions, relapses and exacerbations during 'stress' makes it unwise to use spinal or epidural block. Any persistent postoperative neurological deficit may be blamed on the local anaesthetic, even though there is no reliable confirmatory evidence. There have also been reports· of patients deteriorating after the use of thiopentone but this is discounted by many authorities.

Neuromuscular disorders

Myasthenia gravis, and the myasthenic syndrome which may accompany bronchial carcinoma, resemble partial curarisation. Patients with myasthenia gravis are abnormally sensitive to competitive blocking muscle relaxants and resistant to suxamethonium, but those with myasthenic syndrome are sensitive to all relaxants. There is sometimes increased sensitivity to central nervous system depressant drugs. Regional anaesthesia avoids the hazards. Small doses of atracurium or vecuronium, now fashionable from their relatively short duration, can be used. If there is any doubt about the adequacy of respiration patients should be ventilated postoperatively.

Dystrophia myotonica is a condition in which any stimulus may cause generalized myotonia (muscle contraction with slow relaxation). These patients are often sensitive to thiopentone, suxamethonium is particularly provocative and competitive blocking relaxants rarely relax the tonic muscles. It is better to use inhalation agents both for induction and to produce muscle relaxation. Cardiomyopathy and difficulty in swallowing may be a hazard in these patients.

Acute intermittent porphyria is an absolute contraindication to the use of barbiturates and in particular to the induction agents thiopentone and methohexitone. The administration of barbiturates will precipitate an attack of pain, paralysis and neuropathy. Etomidate appears to be safe as an induction agent.

Disease of the cardiovascular system

All males over 55 years of age, females over 60, and other patients with a history suggesting cardiac disease should have an preoperative electrocardiogram and have it competently evaluated. Dysrhythmias, signs of myocardial ischaemia, old or new infarcts and signs of alteration in the size of any of the heart chambers are all important.

Sinus dysrhythmia and a varying PR interval ('variable pace-maker') are common, and normal in the young healthy patient.

Sinus bradycardia may slow dangerously further with trich-loroethylene and other vagotonic drugs or vagal stimulation (such as traction on a viscus). Premedication should include atropine (best given 0.3–0.6 mg intravenously immediately before induction). Suxamethonium without prior atropine should be avoided.

Ventricular ectopics may indicate electrolyte abnormalities — particularly hypokalaemia. Ectopics carry a risk of progression to ventricular tachycardia or even fibrillation, and the risk is particularly enhanced by stimulation during light anaesthesia and oral surgery. Pre-operative beta blockade with oral propranolol (10–40 mg every 8 h) or until the ectopics are reduced to an acceptable level (say less than 8 per min) should be considered and lignocaine should be at hand for intravenous administration (1–1.5 mg/kg).

Atrial fibrillation. Digitalis preparations should be employed to control irregular ventricular contractions. Beta blockers can also be used with caution unless there is congestive heart failure.

Heart block. Bifascicular block may change to cardiac standstill if myocardial conductivity and excitability are decreased, as may happen with halogenated anaesthetic agents. The management of the anaesthetic is safer if a temporary or permanent intravenous pacemaker is inserted pre-operatively.

Valvular defects. Cardiac output cannot be readily increased. Techniques which may change heart rate, increase venous return (preload) or increase pulmonary vascular resistance should be avoided. Antibiotic cover must be used, particularly for dental extractions. Amoxycillin is the drug usually employed.

Ischaemic heart disease. The risk of death following anaesthesia and elective surgery within six months of myocardial infarction is unacceptably high, and should not be contemplated unless the dangers of denying surgery are greater.

Any patient who presents with symptoms (angina) or signs (old infarction or S–T segment changes on the electrocardiograph of myocardial ischaemia) should be specially assessed preoperatively by exercise testing to establish the threshold for ischaemic changes. Coronary angiography may be used to establish the nature and site of obstruction to myocardial perfusion. Kinetic studies of ventricular motion may indicate the degree of functional impairment. 'Heavy' premedication is frequently used to reduce the stress on the cardiovascular system from such stimulation as insertion of intravascular lines in the awake patient before anaesthesia is induced. An attempt should be made to reduce heart work with anti-hypertensives and beta blockers, and to improve coronary flow with transcutaneous or sublingual trinitroglycerine (which should be continued during the operation and post-operative period). Calcium channel blocking drugs such as nifedipine may also be useful. Coronary artery bypass grafting may be indicated before other major elective surgery. Everything should be done during anaesthesia to avoid tachycardia, hypotension, increases in blood pressure, or hypoxia.

Congestive heart failure should be treated preoperatively with diuretics. If the patient is already under treatment, long-term diuretics with inadequate potassium replacement may have produced hypokalaemia. The serum potassium should be increased to at least 3.5 mmol/l by oral potassium supplements or, if time is short, by slow intravenous infusion with electrocardiographic monitoring. Do not give more than 10 mmol of potassium chloride per h.

Hypertension is common by middle age. Blood pressure greater than 150 mmHg systolic or 100 mmHg diastolic should usually be treated pre-operatively.

The aim should be to bring blood pressure down to the normal range before undertaking elective surgery. Mild cases (systolic 150–175 mmHg, diastolic 100–110 mmHg) can be treated with thiazide diuretics, and potassium supplement with or without addition of beta blockers (e.g. propranolol) until control is achieved. Sedatives, (e.g. diazepam) may help to reduce stress induced hypertension. Moderate hypertension (systolic 175–200 mmHg, diastolic 110–130 mmHg with retinal vessel changes) is managed with antihypertensive drugs like captopril; the dosage being gradually increased until control is achieved. Severe hypertension systolic greater than 200 mmHg or diastolic greater than 140 mmHg with severe retinopathy) should be treated as an emergency in an intensive care ward with continuous or rapid mechanical measurement of arterial pressure available. Hydralazine (5–20 mg intravenously) repeated every hour is the first line of treatment. Labetalol (20–50 mg) or propranolol (1–5 mg) intravenously are indicated if the hypertension fails to respond, and should begin with an infusion of dilute nitroprusside or nitroglycerine, using continuous intra-arterial monitoring of blood presure. The possibility of undiagnosed phaeochromocytoma should be considered.

Respiratory disease

Acute respiratory tract infections such as coryza, sore throat, tonsillitis, largyngitis, tracheitis, acute bronchitis, or pneumonia should signal the postponement of elective surgery until the patient has recovered. Antibiotics may be indicated. The risk of delaying emergency surgery must be weighed against that of the surgical pathology becoming worse.

Chronic respiratory infection should be treated with the appropriate antibiotics and bronchodilators, and by chest physiotherapy to clear retained secretions. Repeated simple lung function tests should be used to monitor improvement. Smoking should be prohibited and regional anaesthetic techniques (intercostal block, thoracic or lumbar epidural block, subarachnoid block etc.) should be considered. They may save the patient from general anaesthesia, improve his ability to cough and eliminate the need for postoperative respiratory depressant analgesics.

Asthma and bronchospasm. A history of wheezing may be related to drug allergy, exercise, stress, emotion, or be seasonal. Provocative factors should be eliminated. Simple pulmonary function tests should be done, and specifically the forced expiratory volume in one second (FEVI) before and after bronchodilators. The patient's most effective bronchodilator should be given immediately preoperatively. Premedication with steroids (hydrocortisone 100 mg intramuscularly) or antihistamines (promethazine 50 mg intramuscularly) with atropine (0.6 mg) may reduce likelihood of bronchospasm. Unnecessary tracheal intubation should be avoided and known bronchodilating agents, especially halothane, or isoflurane and enflurane should be used. Narcotic analgesics (morphine, and omnopon) certain muscle relaxants, for example (suxamethonium, d-tubocurarine, and alcuronium) and propranolol may release histamine and provoke or worsen bronchospasm. An etomidate, vecuronium, fentanyl and halothane sequence is one of the most benign combinations for the anaesthetic management of this condition.

Anaesthetists should be cautious about labelling intraoperative bronchospasm as an allergic phenomenon. It is more likely to have been precipitated by the inhalation of an irritant and may indicate aspiration of gastric contents, a kinked tracheal tube or a foreign body in the airway. If the tube has entered one main bronchus, the signs may mimic severe bronchospasm.

Abdominal conditions

Hiatus hernia, an oesophageal pouch, reflux oesophagitis, haematemesis, intestinal obstruction, and pregnancy near term are all conditions which increase the risk of aspiration pneumonitis. Preoperative precautions to reduce gastric acidity should be employed (see Chapter 11). For example, ranitidine (150 mg 6 hourly for 2 doses), sodium citrate (30 ml 0.3 molar) at induction and the use of rapid sequence intubation technique or regional anaesthetic techniques should be considered.

Preoperative oxygen by face mask on the ward may reduce gaseous abdominal distension in intestinal obstruction as nitrogen in the gut will be replaced by oxygen and absorbed into the bloodstream.

Liver failure

Liver failure has a number of implications for the anaesthetist:-

1. *Impaired drug metabolism.* The metabolism of some drugs, including barbiturates, benzodiazepines and lignocaine,

will be slowed down. Smaller doses of these drugs should be used and titrated with care.

2. *Failure of synthesis of protein*, to which some drugs become strongly bound in plasma, releases more free drug and results in enhanced action. Reduced dose of these drugs should be given or drugs unaffected by protein binding (atracurium for example) should be chosen.

3. *Reduced suxamethonium breakdown* occurs because less plasma pseudocholinesterase is produced in the liver and suxamethonium apnoea may result. Suxamethonium should therefore be avoided or if necessary a peripheral nerve stimulator should be used to monitor the effect of cautious, small doses.

4. *Hepatotoxicity*. Halogenated anaesthetics are variously metabolised in the liver (halothane 15–20%, enflurane 2% and isoflurane 0.2%). The metabolites of halothane have been blamed for so called 'halothane-hepatitis', as a result of which perhaps 1 in 35,000 patients develops massive hepatic necrosis. Other factors are believed to be: repeated halothane anaesthesia, relative or actual hypoxia, or hypotension during anaesthesia. The signs of subclinical postoperative hepatitis after halothane anaesthesia include unexplained jaundice, fever, anorexia, arthralgia or weight loss. Malignancy, radiotherapy, female gender, middle-age obesity, gall bladder disease, thyrotoxicosis, enzyme induction, or a familial tendency may be additional factors which enhance the risk. Children under eight years seem, so far, largely to have escaped this rare condition.

   The British Committee on the Safety of Medicines recommend that it is prudent to avoid repeated halothane anaesthesia within three months, especially if any of the above conditions applies, unless there is a specific indication.

5. *A reduction of clotting factors* (fibrinogen, prothrombin,

factors V, VII, IX and X) which are produced in the liver may occur in liver failure and result in an increased haemorrhagic tendency.

Vitamin K absorption is reduced if there is biliary stasis and so impaired clotting with a prolonged prothrombin time may result. Vitamin K (10–20 mg intramuscularly) should be given pre-operatively.

Hypersplenism with increased consumption of platelets may accompany portal hypertension. Platelet transfusion or fresh blood may be necessary.

If clotting is impaired and not readily remediable, epidural cannulation is best avoided, because of the risk of causing an expanding epidural haematoma which may compress the spinal cord. Other instrumentation, e.g. nasal intubation, may also provoke excessive bleeding.

Operations on the liver often result in massive blood loss. Several large gauge intravenous cannulae should be inserted. Central venous and pulmonary artery wedge pressure should be used together with observation of urine output to monitor fluid balance and cardiac performance.

Hepatorenal failure (renal failure secondary to liver failure) has an obscure origin but it may be due to the failure of the liver to remove vasoactive substances. Adequate hydration, promotion of diuresis by osmotic agents (mannitol), or frusemide reduce the risk.

Renal disease

Many drugs are partly excreted by the kidneys. The muscle relaxant gallamine is entirely excreted in this way and is best avoided in severe renal failure. There is less concern about the potentially adverse renal effect of the fluoride ion, the principal metabolic product of enflurane, than was the case with the now defunct agent methoxyflurane. Halothane or isoflurane are suitable alternatives.

The excretion of nondepolarizing relaxants, neostigmine, atropine, digoxin, and aminoglycoside antibiotics depends on renal function, and doses should be reduced in renal failure. Other drugs do not depend solely on renal excretion and are usually safe; they include inhalational anaesthetics, local anaesthetics, ketamine, etomidate, barbiturates, propofol, droperidol, phenothiazines, benzodiazepines, and non-depolarizing muscle relaxants.

Anaemia is chronic and common, due to the depression of erythopoiesis by uraemia. It is better to accept it rather than to risk cardiac failure from overtransfusion, but the inspired oxygen concentration during anaesthesia should be 40% or more.

Hyperkalemia (potassium more than 5.5 mmol/l is common. Diuretics may reduce the level; if not, insulin 20 units with glucose 20 g intravenously cause rapid fall in plasma potassium as the potassium ion is driven into the cells by insulin.

Endocrine disease

Hyperthyroidism is a potentially dangerous condition. All hyperthyroid patients should be made euthyroid preoperatively, except in a dire emergency, by the administration of Lugol's iodine and beta-blockers. Surgical bleeding may be troublesome. Postoperative wound haematoma occasionally causes respiratory obstruction in the early postoperative period.

Hypothyroidism is an indication for preoperative substitution therapy. Cardiomyopathy and dysrhythmias may occur.

Phaeochromocytoma can pose considerable problems for the anaesthetist. Oversecretion of catecholamines causes severe hypertension with the secondary effects of tachycardia and cardiomyopathy.

Preoperative management begins about two weeks before

surgery with hospitalisation. Alpha-adrenergic blockade is achieved by the administration of phenoxybenzamine, after which increasing doses of beta-adrenergic blockers (propranolol up to 150 mg orally daily) are given until the raised blood pressure and heart rate are controlled to the extent that there is minimal postural hypotension. Blood transfusion or intravenous fluids may be needed to fill the reexpanded vascular space. Intraoperative management is directed to maintaining cardiovascular stability, if necessary with intravenous infusions of vasodilators (nitroprusside or nitroglycerine) or ephedrine. Continuous intravascular blood pressure monitoring is mandatory.

Adrenal cortical hypofunction (Addison's disease) is an indication for the use of supplementary steroids. Hydrocortisone 100 mg intramuscularly or intravenously at induction is satisfactory for short lasting body surface surgery. For major procedures, hydrocortisone 100 mg is given six hourly intravenously until the patient can take oral cortisone acetate postoperatively (25 mg six hourly). A patient with otherwise unexplained hypotension on steroids should immediately be given hydrocortisone 100 mg intravenously.

Adrenal hyperfunction (Cushing's syndrome) and prolonged use of steroids result in electrolyte disturbances, osteoporosis, hypertension, obesity and fragile veins . Neck X-rays reveal the extent of the cervical osteoporosis, with risk of spinal cord damage and potential difficulty in intubation.

Diabetes complicates anaesthesia because starvation means that carbohydrate intake and oral medications may be withheld. Postoperative nausea, vomiting and inability to take in oral sustenance may cause the loss of diabetic control, and the clinical signs of hypo or hyperglycaemia may, confusingly, resemble those of general anaesthesia.

The regimen chosen for the management of the diabetic depends on the severity of the diabetes, the normal method of control and the nature of the operation. The objective is to keep blood sugar as near normal as possible, but hypo-glycaemia is more dangerous than hyperglycaemia. Oral glucose should never be given before anaesthesia, as hypertonic solutions in the stomach increase the risk of vomiting and aspiration and are not absorbed.

1. *Well controlled diabetics for trivial, body surface surgery* are easily managed. A suitable plan is to arrange for surgery about 4 hours after the last meal. 5% dextrose 500 ml is infused over 4 h intravenously and the usual anti-diabetic regimen is maintained whilst monitoring blood glucose each hour by finger stick testing.

2. *Orally-controlled diabetics for major surgery*. Omit antidiabetic therapy one half life before operation (chlorpropamide 48 hours, glibenclamide — on the morning of the operation) and maintain the usual carbohydrate intake. Blood sugar is measured by the finger stick method one hour preoperatively and two hourly thereafter. Five percent dextrose or 0.9% saline are given as required to keep the blood glucose in the normal range of 5–10 mmol/l. Oral therapy begins when oral food intake is reestablished. If the patient's blood sugar exceeds the normal range, a change should be made to a intravenous insulin-glucose-potassium regimen, (see below).

3. *Insulin dependent diabetics undergoing elective major surgery, or emergency surgery in any diabetic*. A baseline blood sugar is estimated by the finger stick method and a specimen is sent to the laboratory for comparison. A solution containing 10 mmol of potassium chloride and 10 units of Actrapid insulin in 500 ml of 5% dextrose is prepared and set up as an infusion with a giving set which includes a 100 ml burette. One hundred ml of solution is given each hour. Blood sugar estimations are made every hour and Actrapid insulin is added according to the sliding scale indicated in Table 12.1.

Table 12.1 Scheme for the addition of Actrapid soluble insulin to an infusion of 5% dextrose at the rate of 100 ml per h to which 2 units of Actrapid insulin and 2 mmols of potassium chloride per 100 ml have already been added

Blood glucose measurement (mmol/litre)	Urine glucose (approx)	Additional Actrapid Soluble insulin (units)
Less than 5		Nil
5 to 7		1
8 to 10	1%	2
11 to 20		3
More than 20	2%	4

Oral carbohydrates and subcutaneous insulin are started again when oral intake is resumed. Urinalysis is only of historical interest now that simple ward blood tests are available.

General considerations in diabetes. Above all, avoid hypoglycaemia. Complications of diabetes may necessitate anaesthesia and surgery, and cause blindness, retinopathy, peripheral neuropathy, autonomic dystrophy, peripheral vascular disease and myocardial ischaemia. Tourniquets should not be used.

Diabetics are prone to infection. Asepsis should be exemplary.

Haematology

Anaemia It is a general rule (except when surgery is necessary to control bleeding) in the United Kingdom and the USA that if the preoperative haemoglobin is less then 10 g/dl, elective surgery (in which bleeding is expected) should not be undertaken until the anaemia is corrected and its cause is clear. Anaemia results in decreased oxygen supply to tissues, reduced reserve of oxygen if hypoxia occurs, and poor ability to tolerate blood loss. High output cardiac failure can also occur.

Anaemia should be corrected medically (if this is feasible in the time available before surgery) or by blood transfusion. It should be remembered that it takes all of 24 h for oxygen carriage by stored blood to reach normal values (because it is deficient in 2–3 diphosphoglycerate (2–3 DPG), the enzyme responsible for delivery of oxygen to the tissues) and to allow the cardiovascular system to readjust after the additional blood is given.

Excessive destruction of red blood cells may require splenectomy, e.g. in spherocytosis. Blood transfusion is generally withheld until the spleen is removed, to prevent destruction of the transfused red cells.

Chronic anaemia, as in renal failure, or among undernourished populations in developing countries, is reasonably well tolerated by both the patient and anaesthetist because of compensatory production of 2–3 DPG. Indeed, blood transfusion may suppress further red cell production and precipitate congestive cardiac failure — as one of the authors found out the hard way when working in a developing country.

Sickle cell disease and sickle cell trait. All patients of African, Caribbean, Asian, Middle Eastern or Mediterranean origin are potentially at risk from sickle cell problems from a gene which produces abnormal haemoglobin. A test known as the Sickledex® test is useful for screening patients. It will determine whether the patient has the abnormal sickling gene but it will not distinguish whether he is suffering from the dangerous homozygous sickle cell disease or the milder heterozygous sickle cell trait. The red cells in the homozygous sickle cell become sickleshaped when provoked by hypoxia or acidosis: stasis is produced by the sickled cells obstructing blood flow and the 'vicious, viscous sickle cycle' results.

Infarction of distal tissue then occurs, obviously catastrophic if vital organs are affected.

These complications can be lessened if the anaesthetist knows beforehand. The risks are reduced by preoxygenation, high inspired oxygen during anaesthesia, mechanical hyperventilation which also increases pH, haemodilution with intravenous crystalloid solutions (or dextran 40) to reduce viscosity, and postoperative added oxygen. Tourniquets are forbidden because of the danger of thrombosis. Exchange transfusion may be necessary preoperatively before major surgery.

Patients with heterozygous sickle cell trait are much less likely to suffer sickling crises but should be managed as for sickle cell disease.

Haemophilia varies considerably in severity. Liaison with the local haemophilia centre usually ensures that the patient is given appropriate clotting factor replacement in time to prevent excessive operative bleeding. Anything which may increase bleeding is avoided.

Thrombocytopenia. Preoperative and intraoperative platelet transfusion is necessary before major surgery if platelet count is less than 100,000. Continuous epidural block is contraindicated because of the risk of producing an expanding epidural haematoma which may cause spinal cord damage.

Surgery during pregnancy

Surgery for concurrent conditions should be avoided if possible especially in the first trimester. Although there is no proven correlation between anaesthesia and fetal malformation or impairment, surgery may precipitate an abortion. If anaesthesia is essential, local anaesthesia should be considered and only well tried drugs known to have minimal ill effects should be used for general anaesthesia.

There is increased risk to the mother as a patient in later pregnancy. The stomach contents are more acid and the risk of aspiration is increased. The supine hypotension syndrome may place the fetus at risk, and drugs given at delivery may depress the neonate and relax the uterus, possibly causing increased haemorrhage (Chapter 10).

In toxaemia of pregnancy general anaesthesia is sometimes preferred to epidural or spinal block, to reduce the risks of wild swings in blood pressure — associated with sympathetic blockade in the presence of a reduced circulating blood volume.

Obesity

Gross obesity can be defined as anything above an additional 50% of the patient's ideal weight (roughly: in kg, height in cm −100 for men and −105 in females). The condition is difficult to cure and presents many problems to the anaesthetist — not least, the weighty problem of moving, lifting or positioning the patient (surgeons always seem to be 'scrubbed up' or drinking coffee when there is a patient to be lifted.) There is also an increased risk of regurgitation, intubation difficulties, inaccessibility of veins, inadequacy of noninvasive blood pressure measurement, and postoperative respiratory failure from the weight of fat of the anterior abdominal wall. Postoperatively there is an increased likelihood of deep vein thrombosis and pulmonary embolism. Thoracic epidural blockade with general anaesthesia has advantages over conventional general anaesthesia so far as postoperative respiratory function is concerned, but there may be considerable mechanical difficulties in placing the catheter.

Doses of drugs should be based on lean body mass, not on whole body weight, and are better given intravenously than through needles too short to reach muscle.

Old age

Old age brings with it an accummulation of complicating conditions. The preoperative evaluation of any patient over 65 years must include haemoglobin, urea or creatinine and electrolyte estimation, chest X-ray and ECG. Admission to the ward two days preoperatively, for all but the most healthy and active, provides time for observation and investigation and gives the elderly patient time to adjust to unfamiliar surroundings.

Anaesthesia has a reputation for causing prolonged confusion in the elderly. There is some truth in this, and certainly older patients operated on for cataracts under local anaesthesia are less likely to be disorientated than those given general anaesthesia. But the social disruption, pain after surgery, and the effects of hospitalisation also contribute. It is wise to use atropine rather than hyoscine for premedication as hyoscine certainly causes confusion in the elderly. Limited doses of pethidine or morphine may be given if they are indicated, but only small doses of central nervous system depressant drugs should be used, carefully titrated against response.

Fragile bones and loss of muscle mass make the elderly more susceptible to trauma on the operating table. Elderly patients tolerate operations under local anaesthesia excellently. Regional blockade is particularly valuable for such common procedures as transurethal prostatectomy or repair of fractured hip, but spinal osteoarthritis makes its administration technically more difficult. An analgesic dose of ketamine (0.5 mg/kg) greatly eases discomfort during the establishing of spinal subarachnoid or epidural anaesthesia. If general anaesthesia is chosen, the elderly require, and deserve, extra care because of their increased vulnerability to every complication or hazard.

13

Complications and hazards

First woman: 'Did you have gas for your operation?'
Second woman: 'No, they don't give you gas any more. A bloke comes and sticks a needle in the back of your hand four or five times, and then you go off to sleep.'
World Medicine, 5 March, 1983

Patients accept that an operation will result in discomfort and pain, and that surgical complications may arise. Such complications are tolerated as inevitable providing they are only temporary. The hazards of anaesthesia, and the skill which the anaesthetist must sometimes display to avoid them and their consequences, are often less well understood or appreciated. Questions from patients such as 'do you stay with me throughout the operation after giving me the injection?' or, in private practice, 'Why do I have to pay so much to the anaesthetist just for an injection in the arm?' are not unknown even at the present time. This chapter outlines some of the hazards of anaesthesia, both predictable and unpredictable, of which the unconscious patient under anaesthesia may be blissfully unaware.

The major hazards of anaesthesia have many causes. Some of these are initially trivial, but if they are unrecognised, or are badly managed, catastrophe may result. Other hazards may not be disastrous but are major sources of discomfort, pain, or irritation to the patient. The complications of local anaesthetic agents and techniques of local anaesthesia were considered in Chapter 9.

Deaths 'under' or 'due to' anaesthesia

'Death under anaesthesia' may not necessarily be 'due to anaesthesia' or its complications. If massive uncontrollable haemorrhage occurs during surgery it is certainly a 'death under anaesthesia' but it is not a death 'due to anaesthesia' — although the anaesthetist has had an important role to play in attempting to keep the patient alive by attending to the rapid transfusion of blood.

Potential lethal anaesthetic hazards

Deaths *due* to anaesthesia are fortunately rare in anaesthetically developed countries — possible one per 100,000 anaesthetics in the United Kingdom. When such a death does occur, the two most likely causes (hypoxia and cardiac arrest) are interrelated; in both cases death is due to the brain and/or the heart being deprived of oxygen either primarily (caused by respiratory hypoxia) or secondarily (as the result of circulatory standstill following cardiac arrest). Other, fortunately less common, potentially fatal hazards due to anaesthesia are acute anaphylaxis to drugs used in anaesthesia, and malignant hyperthermia.

Respiratory hypoxia or anoxia during anaesthesia

The terms 'hypoxia' and 'anoxia' are often loosely used interchangeably but, strictly speaking, 'hypoxia' means 'diminished', and 'anoxia' total, deprivation of oxygen from the tissues.

Hypoxia or anoxia during anaesthesia due to respiratory

failure results from the partial or total failure or obstruction of the supply of oxygen to the brain. This can occur at any point between the source of supply of oxygen, through the anaesthetic machine and the upper and lower respiratory passages of the patient, the lungs and major blood vessels, to the capillaries and ultimately the transfer of oxygen to and within the cells. Most other tissues will recover from hypoxia (or even anoxia) lasting many minutes, but the brain becomes irretrievably damaged after 4 to 6 min deprivation of oxygen, as will occur if the heart stops beating effectively (cardiac arrest).

Failure of the oxygen supply to the anaesthetic apparatus may be due to:

1. Exhaustion of the oxygen supply (if cylinders are allowed to empty for example).
2. Disconnection, cross-connection or interruption of the oxygen pipeline[1].

The anaesthetist must ensure:

1. That if pipelines are used, they are properly and securely attached to the anaesthetic machine. The valve of the oxygen cylinder supplying the machine is opened and that the cylinder contains oxygen if cylinders are used.
2. That oxygen is reaching the anaesthetic machine from the source of supply and being delivered at the patient outlet. Modern machines are equipped with oxygen analysers which indicate the percentage of oxygen delivered and sound the alarm if it is not high enough.
3. That reserve cylinders are full and that a key is available to open them.

---

[1] Present day anaesthetists in anaesthetically developed countries too easily regard the oxygen supply from the pipes from the wall or boom oxygen outlet as accurately labelled and inexhaustable. Deaths have occurred from crossed oxygen and nitrous oxide pipelines even in recent years. In another incident a mechanical digger summarily severed the oxygen supply to the whole of a major teaching hospital.

4. That all oxygen alarms are functioning before the anaesthetic is started.
5. That the oxygen supply gauges continue to indicate that
   the supply is adequate throughout the anaesthetic. If
   cylinders are being used, constant vigilance is required to
   ensure that cylinders do not empty unnoticed. Modern
   anaesthetic machines are fitted with alarms and devices to
   cut off the nitrous oxide supply in the event of oxygen
   failure and air entrainment devices, but dangerous hypoxia
   may supervene before these are activated.

Failure of the oxygen delivery system to the patient may be due
to:
1. Leaks at various points in the apparatus.
2. Disconnection of the machine from the patient. This is
   particularly dangerous if the patient is paralysed with a
   muscle relaxant and breathing is maintained artificially.
   Alarms are normally fitted nowadays but they are usually
   activated by a fall in airway pressure and are therefore of
   little use when the patient is breathing spontaneously.

   If malfunction of the apparatus is suspected it should
   be disconnected from the patient, even if this causes the
   patient to wake up. If the patient is paralysed and a second
   machine is not immediately available, a hand operated self-
   expanding resuscitation bag should be used, and should
   be part of the equipment of all operating theatres.

Failure to intubate the patient is another cause of hypoxia.
No one can guarantee to intubate the larynx — even experienced anaesthetists admit that on occasion they cannot.
Preoperative assessment of the patient's upper airway
anatomy may warn of potential difficulty, but the most
careful examination may fail. If the first attempt to intubate
a patient fails it is important not to persist vainly and cause
trauma and rapidly progressive hypoxia. It is far better to
revert to mask ventilation, reassess the situation and devise
a means of solving the problem, either by using a technique

that does not require intubation, or with different laryngo-scopes, introducers or tubes, while help is summoned. If there is a risk of regurgitation of stomach contents, pressure should be applied to the cricoid cartilage to obstruct the oesophagus (Sellick's manoeuvre (Chapter 11) and the patient turned on to the left side, head down until respiration and protective reflexes return.

The golden rules are:-

1. Never paralyse a patient you cannot ventilate. This is easier said than done. Cautious anaesthetists ventilate elective patients after administering the induction agent but before giving the muscle relaxant, but this is a dangerous practice if the patient is suspected of having a full stomach.

2. Always have an alternative means of ventilating a patient readily available in case of apparatus failure, but otherwise use an anaesthetic face mask (preferably with an oropharyngeal airway to keep the tongue forward and the airway unobstructed). Expired air respiration (EAR) is the last resource, this need not be directly mouth-to-mouth or mouth-to-nose respiration; an anaesthetic mask, again preferably with an airway in place, is an excellent device for administering EAR (Chapter 14).

3. Be trained and prepared for the rare occasion when there is irretrievable total obstruction of the upper airway. Emergency tracheotomy is a hazardous procedure but the cricothyroid membrane is superficial and all medical, nursing and experienced paramedical personnel should be prepared at least to pierce it with a wide bore needle or cannula (12 g or larger) to provide a minimal airway (Chapter 11).

Accidental oesophageal intubation is fatally easy, and not always recognised. A 'burping' noise on inflation may be the clue. Failure to produce a sound from the tube if the chest is smartly compressed or the absence of expired carbon dioxide (if an analyser is available) will confirm the misplacement. Cyanosis is a poor early sign, as it may be slow to develop if the patient has been preoxygenated and the anaesthetist may be deceived into thinking that all is well.

Mechanical obstruction in the gas delivery system can occur anywhere along its length. The cause may be simple — for example when the surgeon's elbow may be firmly planted on an anaesthetic tube — or less obviously when, for instance, the cuff of a tracheal tube herniates over the end, or the tracheal tube has not been checked before use and a foreign body has forced its way into the lumen[2].

Mechanical obstruction in the spontaneously breathing patient results in:

1. An increase in the effort needed by the patient to inspire.
2. Paradoxical movement of the chest and abdomen, which rise and fall alternately.
3. An indrawing of intercostal and supraclavicular spaces.
4. 'Tugging' of the trachea and larynx at each breath.
5. Distension of the reservoir bag if the expiratory valve is closed or the scavenging system is obstructed or not functioning properly. Such situations are highly dangerous and can lead to rupture of the lung — 'pop-off' safety valves are usually provided.
6. Progressive cyanosis.
7. Tachycardia followed by bradycardia and ultimately cardiac arrest and death.

[2] Descriptions of frightening episodes of obstruction from foreign bodies in endotracheal tubes are among the most frequent submitted to the editors of correspondence columns of anaesthesia journals. The foreign bodies responsible have included dead cockroaches, tapeworms, ampoule and suction union tops, and metal diaphragms left by the manufacturers in new connectors. Tracheal tubes and their connections should be closely inspected before insertion. The use of an introducer passed through the lumen of the connector and tube is a useful precaution as well as an aid to intubation.

Mechanical obstruction in the patient who is on controlled ventilation is usually manifest by difficulty or failure to inflate the chest when the reservoir bag is squeezed, and progressive cyanosis, tachycardia, bradycardia and death if a solution to the problem is not forthcoming.

Obstruction due to bronchospasm is more likely to occur in patients who are known to be asthmatic or smokers. It may be provoked by tracheal intubation, tracheal suction, irritant anaesthetic agents (ether, trichloroethylene, isoflurane, etc), an anaphylactoid response, respiratory infection, inhalation of stomach contents, surgical stimulation or movement of the tracheal tube during light anaesthesia.

Less frequently, drugs may release histamine and cause bronchospasm. Tubocurarine and some other muscle relaxants, gelatine plasma expanders, dextran and cremophor EL — used as a solubilizer — have all been implicated.

Bronchospasm may be recognised by wheezing, signs of hypoxia and hypercarbia. In the ventilated patient, higher than normal inflation pressure is needed.

Hypoxia due to cardiovascular causes may be from cardiac or vascular abnormalities including arteriovenous shunts, one lung anaesthesia, low cardiac output states, hypovolaemic shock from blood or fluid loss, pulmonary oedema, or impaired venous return from pressure by over zealous surgical retraction.

The treatment of respiratory obstruction

The principle of the treatment of mechanical obstruction in the anaesthetic system is to eliminate the cause. Numerous descriptions in the journals demonstrate that the first automatic reaction of an anaesthetist who is unable to ventilate a patient is to assume that the cause of the difficulty is bronchospasm, especially if he has just passed a tracheal tube that he believes has a patent lumen. This can be a fatal error.

A differential diagnosis between mechanical obstruction and bronchospasm must first be made. Mechanical obstruction is more common and more likely to be total, whereas in bronchospasm wheezing can usually be heard with or without a stethoscope. The cause of the obstruction may be obvious — for example, it may be treatable by simply straightening a kinked tube in the back of the oral cavity. If the tube is placed too far into the trachea, it will usually enter the right main bronchus. This may easily escape notice, especially if a high concentration of oxygen is in use, until signs of hypoxia, hypercarbia or respiratory obstruction become apparent. The complication can be avoided if the anaesthetist checks the position of the tube after insertion by listening with a stethoscope over each side of the chest while manually inflating the lungs — the absence of breath sounds or expansion on one side of the chest is diagnostic, and the tube should be gradually withdrawn until air is heard to enter both sides of the thorax equally. The use of tubes already cut to the right length reduces the risk.

The anaesthetist must never forget that, when faced with inexplicable mechanical obstruction immediately after intubation, the best advice is:

'*When in doubt take it out*'

Mechanical obstruction in the unintubated patient, whether breathing spontaneously or being inflated (for example before intubation) is most often due to the tongue falling back. It can usually be remedied by extending the head, pushing the chin forward and inserting an oral or nasal anaesthetic airway (see Chapter 6, Fig. 6.1).

Mechanical obstruction in the intubated patient may be mystifying. The first essential is to realise that the presence of a tracheal tube does not guarantee a clear airway. The tube can become kinked, its bevel can impinge on the side of the trachea, it may be advanced too far and enter the right main bronchus or the cuff may herniate over the end.

The treatment of bronchospasm

Bronchospasm requires treatment with drugs; but the first essential is to ensure that there is no mechanical obstruction, either anatomical, due to the tongue falling back in the unintubated person, or due to the apparatus defects which have already been mentioned.

Intravenous ephedrine in 5 mg increments intravenously or 30 mg intramuscularly may be helpful but may cause tachycardia and elevate the blood pressure. Alternatively, a slow intravenous injection of aminophylline 5 mg/kg followed by an infusion of 0.5 mg/kg/h may be effective, or a beta adrenergic stimulant such as salbutamol (up to 250 μg slowly as an injection followed by an infusion of 5 μg/min) or terbutaline can be used. Nebulised salbutamol or terbutaline can also be useful. Steroids (hydrocortisone 100 mg intravenously) are used in resistant cases. Prolonged ventilation and neuromuscular block in the Intensive Care Unit may be necessary in the worst cases. Adrenaline 1 ml of 1 : 1000 solution subcutaneously is an effective measure in desperate cases. Dilute infusions of ketamine and ventilation with halothane have also been used successfully.

Cardiac and circulatory arrest

'Cardiac arrest' is a term used for failure of the heart to achieve an adequate output due to standstill (asystole) or dysrhythmias (usually ventricular fibrillation). 'Circulatory arrest' would be a better description of the condition, but 'cardiac arrest' is the term in common use — even when the heart is fibrillating and thus, strictly speaking, not arrested completely.

Cardiac arrest may be secondary to respiratory hypoxia or anoxia, or it may be primarily due to mechanical insults (e.g. pulmonary embolism, cardiac tamponade or gross valvular incompetence) or to lack of circulatory blood volume after haemorrhage.

The principles of the treatment of cardiac or circulatory arrest are the same whether it occurs in the operating theatre or elsewhere, except that in the former it is obviously essential that anaesthetic drugs must be stopped and 100% oxygen substituted for inhaled agents. The treatment of cardiac arrest is described in Chapter 14; in this chapter the treatment of prearrest dysrhythmias will be considered. If dysrhythmias are observed on the electrocardiograph, diagnosed, and effectively dealt with, most potential arrests in the operating theatre will be avoided. Patients who do suffer cardiac arrest in the operating theatre generally stand a better chance of survival than those who arrest elsewhere, especially if they are intubated, because of the ready availability of skilled staff, apparatus and appropriate drugs.

The diagnosis and treatment of cardiac dysrhythmias

Monitoring with the electrocardiograph (ECG) is considered nowadays to be mandatory during anaesthesia. The treatment of dysrhythmias before they become life threatening is of great importance.

Bradycardia 0–40 beats/min is sometimes seen, and not treated in awake, healthy individuals; but if bradycardia develops during an ordinary anaesthetic, a cause must be sought and corrected. If the heart rate continues to slow, like a clock running down, hypoxia is likely to be the cause and should immediately be treated by checking and improving the oxygen supply to the brain.

Surgical stimuli, including pressure on the eyeball (the occulocardiac reflex), traction on the peritoneum, Fallopian tubes or vas deferens, may cause bradycardia by vagal reflexes. A cautionary word should be addressed to the over vigorous surgeon. Intravenous atropine 0.3–1.0 mg will usually resolve the problem.

Halogenated volatile anaesthetic agents (halothane, enflurane or isoflurane) may also cause sinus bradycardia. Reduction of the inspired concentration usually brings an improvement, as does intravenous atropine.

Other drugs may also slow the heart, (e.g. suxamethonium, anticholinesterases (neostigmine), narcotic analgesics (morphine, fentanyl, alfentanil) local anaesthetic drugs and beta-blockers). The newer muscle relaxants (atracurium and vecuronium) do not cause tachycardia, so the other factors which cause bradycardia may have a greater influence than when muscle relaxant drugs with a vagolytic action (pancuronium, gallamine) are used. The treatment is intravenous atropine.

Heart block rarely occurs during anaesthesia; when it does, it is usually from the use of volatile agents. If intravenous atropine fails to raise the heart rate, slow controlled intravenous infusion of dilute isoprenaline 0.5–5.0 μg/min may improve conduction, cardiac contractility and cardiac output. Cardiac pacemaking may be necessary, meanwhile external cardiac massage should maintain an adequate cardiac output.

Nodal bradycardia is probably the commonest cause of a slow heart rate during anaesthesia[3].

Treatment with atropine and reduction of inspired concentration of volatile agents is necesssary if the blood pressure falls. Junctional and nodal rhythms are common and rarely progress to anything more serious. They can happen without apparent provocation when anaesthesia is too light and, paradoxically, when it is too deep. Providing the blood

---

[3] The vigilant student will impress by pointing out the cannon waves in the neck when a nodal dysrhythmia occurs. It results from the atria contracting whilst the tricuspid valve is shut, so that a pulse is seen conducted back along the jugular venous system.

pressure is maintained, active intervention is best avoided — it is more likely to produce a worse rhythm. If the blood pressure is decreased, treatment depends on the rate at which the heart is beating. If the heart rate is fast beta-blockers should be given.

Premature ventricular contractions (PVCs) may occur even in healthy individuals — for instance, they frequently happen in patients having dental extractions under light inhalational anaesthesia without local anaesthetic cover. Adrenaline injected by the surgeon may provoke ventricular dysrhythmias. The risk is reduced if lignocaine is mixed with the solution.

PVCs only become potentially dangerous if they are excessively numerous (say, more than 8/min), multifocal (i.e. each PVC complex differs), or the PVC begins to encroach on the S–T segment. Any of these situations may suddenly switch to fibrillation. If the cause is not immediately remediable — e.g. by withdrawal of a central venous line which is stimulating the ventricle, correcting electrolyte disturbances (particularly hypokalaemia), increasing ventilation if there is hypercarbia, or reducing inappropriate surgical stimulation — lignocaine should be given intravenously to a maximum of 1.5 mg/kg. This will often suppress the ectopic focus. Lignocaine can then be infused at a rate of 2 mg/min to prevent recurrence. Beta-blockers (propranolol or practolol) are the next resort and may need supplementation by procainamide (100–250 mg i.m.). Amiodarone (5 mg/kg infused over 30 min) is also effective.

Premature atrial contractions (PACs) are usually of little importance, but alert the anaesthetist to the possibility of worse dysrhythmias developing. Propranolol may be needed if cardiac output suffers.

Supraventricular tachycardias are rare, and most likely in patients with severe ischaemic heart disease. Cardiac output may fall to the point where there is no effective peripheral perfusion. Neostigmine is often the nearest available effective remedy before beta-blockers, verapamil or electrical cardioversion can be summoned. The pressor agent methoxamine also slows the heart.

Sinus tachycardia is usually benign, and due to: surgical stimulation during light anaesthesia; tracheal intubation; atropine premedication; the administration of enflurane and isoflurane, pancuronium, gallamine, ketamine or beta-adrenergic stimulants; preoperative pyrexia or anxiety. If any of these causes is unlikely, other correctable factors include hypovolaemia and hypercarbia.

If a sinus tachycardia suddenly arises during anaesthesia unassociated with surgical stimulation, you should consider the possibility of it being the first sign of malignant hyperpyrexia, pulmonary embolism or infarction. Tachycardia related to surgical manipulation, especially in the abdomen, may indicate that the surgeon has squeezed an undiagnosed phaeochromocytoma.

Management is based on the likely cause — if anaesthesia is too light, analgesics and/or a higher concentration of inhaled volatile agent is given. Persistent sinus tachycardia, especially if there are signs of impaired myocardial perfusion (depression of the S-T segment on the ECG), can be treated with beta-blockers, titrated against the heart rate.

Atrial fibrillation is often associated with thyrotoxicosis, ischaemic heart disease, or mitral valve disease. It is unlikely to arise *de novo* during anaesthesia. It should be managed with intravenous beta-blockers and digoxin.

Paroxysmal supraventricular tachycardia must be treated. Calcium channel blocking drugs (e.g. verapamil) are probably the best choice but cardioversion may be necessary. Carotid sinus massage may also be effective — but may be dangerous to the patients who are likely to need it because of the risk of dislodging a plaque of atheroma.

Beta-adrenergic blocking drugs are useful in virtually every dysrhythmia. Although propranolol may cause bronchospasm in asthmatic patients, it is usually the most readily available drug. Beta-blockers are contraindicated only if there is brady-cardia, hypoxia, hypovolaemia or congestive heart failure, or high concentrations of volatile anaesthetic agents are in use.

Hypersensitivity reactions

Full blown anaphylactic reactions precipitated by anaesthetic drugs with massive release of histamine are fortunately rare, but when they do occur they are frightening and hazardous. Minor reactions, for example local or general skin wheals are fairly common. It must be remembered that hypersensitivity reactions may occur during anaesthesia and surgery from agents other than anaesthetic drugs (e.g. contrast media and antibiotics).

The anaesthetic drugs which are most likely to initiate hypersensitivity reactions are induction agents, and to a far lesser extent, muscle relaxants. Several promising induction agents (including propanidid and Althesin®) have been with-drawn because the incidence of reactions, though not great (probably 1 in 8000 to 10,000 administrations) was considered to be too high. The currently available induction agents (thio-pentone, methohexitone, ketamine, etomidate and propofol — in descending order of a likelihood of a hypersensitivity reaction) are relatively safe. Thiopentone probably has a hypersensitivity incidence of about 1 in 20,000 but reactions to it are severe. Hypersensitivity reactions to local anaes-thetics are very rare, most of the so-called reactions are found on investigation to arise from overdosage or direct intravas-cular injection; reaction to accompanying adrenaline is also rare.

The first symptoms of hypersensitivity are usually cutaneous flushing round the face and neck, an itching urti-carial rash, or simply a histaminic 'triple' response along a vein. Often the reaction proceeds no further, and there is a suspicion that the reporting of 'reactions' of this kind has at times unfortunately magnified the apparent incidence of dangerous reactions with some drugs, and even unnecessarily led to their withdrawal.

The major aspects of a severe 'triple' reaction are oedema, vasodilatation and bronchospasm. Oedema occurs in varying degrees of severity, especially around the eyelids, but is sometimes widespread. More seriously, glottic oedema may occur, and is dangerous as it may lead to respiratory obstruction and even the need for cricothyrotomy (Chapter 11).

Vasodilation and the leaking of fluid from the capillaries into the interstitial space can lead to tachycardia and dangerous, pulseless, profound hypotension. Bronchospasm can range from a transient difficulty in inflation to status asthmaticus.

Treatment is according to symptomatic severity — the most severe require 100% oxygen and controlled ventilation, the infusion of 1000 ml or more of colloid solution (human albumen solution (HAS), hetastarch (Hespan®), gelatine (Haemaccel®) etc), adrenaline intramuscularly (or with caution intravenously) and intravenous and/or intramuscular hydrocortisone, aminophylline or ephedrine to combat bronchospasm.

Malignant hyperpyrexia

Malignant hyperpyrexia is a potentially fatal inherited defect of muscular metabolism which, when triggered by some drugs, causes a rise of body temperature of at least 2°C per hour accompanied by severe muscle rigidity. If it is not treated, it almost inevitably leads to death from hypoxaemia, metabolic acidosis, hyperkalaemia, hypocalcaemia, acute renal failure and cardiac arrest. The inherited nature of this condition was first brought to light by an Australian report in 1960, though hindsight shows that it had undoubtedly been responsible for a number of earlier unexplained deaths under anaesthesia. Man shares this inherited condition with other animals, including certain species of pigs, which are peculiarly susceptible and useful for research. The triggering agents in man are almost entirely confined to drugs used in anaesthesia; halothane and suxamethonium particularly have been incriminated, though most volatile agents, and even the amide local anaesthetics like lignocaine, have also been implicated.

If the condition occurs, the wary anaesthetist will be alerted by tachycardia, hyperpnoea and cyanosis in addition to hyperpyrexia and muscle rigidity. The inhalation anaesthetic should be immediately withdrawn, 100% oxygen given, respiration controlled, and ice packs used in an attempt to control the temperature rise. The metabolic acidosis is treated with sodium bicarbonate. Insulin may be required for the hyperkalaemia. The specific therapy is dantrolene, which controls cellular calcium distribution to the muscle sarcoplasma. Dantrolene (1 mg/kg) is given by repeated intravenous injection. It may also be given orally prophylactically to suspected potential cases. Many operating theatres keep 'malignant hyperpyrexia kits' in the refrigerator.

Hypotension

Blood pressure (BP) recording is one of the most common forms of monitoring during anaesthesia because it is so easily measured, but undue faith is often put on its value. An unanaesthetised fit young patient (e.g. an injured motor cyclist) can lose between 20 to 40% of his blood volume before his blood pressure falls — because of compensating vasoconstriction. As soon as he is anaesthetised, his blood pressure will fall precipitously due to vasodilation, pooling of blood peripherally, reduced venous return and so decreased cardiac output. He may risk damage to the organs from under perfusion and then suffer cardiac arrest from reduced coronary perfusion.

Perfusion of the tissues is more important than blood pressure. A fit oxygenated patient who while anaesthetised has a BP of 120 mm Hg 'may quite safely be maintained at a BP of 70 to 80 mm Hg under anaesthesia — the volume of oxygenated blood delivered to a unit of tissue may actually be increased due to vasodilation.

Hypotension can result from:

1. *Decreased circulating blood volume* because of inadequate replacement of fluid losses due to dehydration or excessive vomiting, polyuria, ascites, or from fistulae (electrolytes), acute haemorrhage (whole blood) or burns (colloid plasma proteins). Such losses are sometimes described as loss of 'preload'.

2. *Reduced venous return* from raised intrathoracic pressure due to: positive pressure artificial ventilation; pneumothorax; vena caval compression in supine, pregnant patients; gross obesity; abdominal tumours and over vigorous surgical retraction. All these are further examples of inadequate preloading.

3. *Decreased peripheral vascular resistance* from vasodilator drugs — e.g. nitroprusside, alpha-adrenergic blockers, volatile inhalational agents, histamine release or vasodilating techniques (e.g. spinal or epidural block). This may be called reduced 'afterload'.

4. *Impaired myocardial contractility* from drugs (inhalational agents, beta-blockers, myocardial ischaemia, and central nervous system depressants, including all general anaesthetics (except ether), ketamine and etomidate, and high blood levels of local anaesthetics following the injection of large volumes or accidental intravenous injection.

Hypotension is managed by:

1. Restoring the circulating blood volume by an appropriate

infusion of fluid (crystalloid, colloid, or blood). Replacement of haemoglobin is of less importance than the restoration of the intravascular blood volume, particularly if oxygen is administered. Colloid solutions may be used, either by natural blood products (human albumen solution (HAS) or artificial expanders (dextrans, gelatins and starch products — e.g. Dextran® 70, Haemaccel® and Hespan®).

2. Increased oxygenation by raising inspired oxygen and increasing minute ventilation if the ventilation is controlled. If sudden hypotension has occurred it is important to check that hypoxia itself has not caused the fall in blood pressure.

3. Searching for a surgical cause for the fall in blood pressure, and remedying it.

4. Increasing contraction of the myocardium if it is impaired; inotropic drugs, (ephedrine, up to 30 mg, should be given slowly intravenously into a reliable infusion).

5. Avoiding vasopressors such as metaraminol unless there is known peripheral vasodilatation (e.g. due to subarachnoid spinal anaesthesia) as they cause vasoconstriction and so reduce tissue perfusion. In a desperate situation, however, they can be used to maintain BP and hence coronary and cerebral circulation while circulatory blood volume is replaced.

Hypertension

Hypertension which develops during anaesthesia may result from:

1. *Tracheal intubation and laryngoscopy*. These manoeuvres commonly cause increased blood pressure. Adequate doses of induction agents, analgesics, intravenous or topical lignocaine, beta-blockers and vasodilators (e.g. nitroprusside and nitroglycerine) may all lessen this effect.

2. *Drugs which produce hypertension*. These include

pancuronium, ketamine, gallamine and excessive doses of inotropic drugs.

3. *Hypercarbia*. This may result from obstruction or depression of respiration or inadequate artificial ventilation. A careful check of the anaesthetic system and measurement of the minute ventilaton should identify the cause. The growing use of carbon dioxide meters to measure expired carbon dioxide will reduce the possibility of unrecognised hypercarbia.

4. *Surgical manipulation* during inadequate anaesthesia can cause hypertension and tachycardia. The anaesthetist must consider whether there is a misconnexion in the system, an empty vaporiser, or a pathological cause, such as an undiagnosed phaeochromocytoma.

5. *Overtransfusion* is easily recognised if central venous pressure monitoring is in use. Signs of congestive failure — frothy sputum in the tracheal tube or reduced compliance — may develop later. The administration of intravenous diuretics (frusemide 5–40 mg) will promote a diuresis, and usually rapidly solve the problem; it is important to catheterise the patient's bladder when these drugs are administered.

The inhalation of stomach contents

This is one of the most dreaded complications of anaesthesia. The respiratory and alimentary tracts cross one another in the pharynx and so gut contents can enter the respiratory tract if the normal protective reflexes are abolished or reduced by general anaesthesia, sedation or loss of consciousness from, for example, head injury or drug overdose. The prevention of inhalation of stomach contents and its treatment is described in Chapter 11.

Hiccoughs

This may be provoked by heavy handed surgeons pulling on structures near the diaphragm, some drugs (e.g. methohexitone) or dilatation of the stomach from gases mistakenly blown down the oesophagus. The treatment is to enhance the neuromuscular block with more relaxant and to deepen anaesthesia.

Iatrogenic trauma

The processes which allow a patient to withstand the elective assaults of the surgeon's knife also render him vulnerable to accidental assault by the anaesthetist and the environment of the operating theatre.

Sore throat. At least 10%, and up to 80% of intubated patients in some series, complain of sore throat with or without hoarseness after tracheal intubation. The incidence depends on a number of factors including the trauma of insertion, the duration of intubation, the type of tube (red rubber tubes are more irritant than the modern disposable plastic variety), the use of local anaesthetic sprays or ointment, and drying drugs such as atropine. Curiously, there is also an incidence of sore throat (sometimes as high as 25%) in patients who have not been intubated, or even had an oropharyngeal airway inserted.

Loss or damage to teeth. Such accidents are probably the most frequent cause of litigation against anaesthetists. If the teeth and gums are unhealthy there is a risk that teeth can be loosened by pressure from the laryngoscope during intubation. Prosthetic teeth, e.g. crowns, are less strong than normal teeth and are particularly vulnerable. The greatest fear is that a tooth or tooth fragment might be inhaled into the lungs. If there is a possibility that this has happened, chest X-rays should be taken and the tooth or fragment removed urgently by bronchoscopy (or even open lung operation if it is otherwise inaccessible).

Pressure lesions on the patient's face. Failure to support the patient's head adequately — especially when turned into the lateral position — may be responsible. Prolonged mask anaesthesia may leave a bruise from anaesthetist's fingers along the line of the jaw — a temporary and mildly uncomfortable occurrence. Vigorous manipulation of the neck may cause nerve damage, particularly if there are arthritic changes. Fracture dislocation may occur, and even damage to the cervical spinal cord. Patients who present with a possible neck injury should only be moved while traction is applied.

Nerve damage may result from compression or stretching of a nerve. The commonest lesions encountered are ulnar nerve palsy (from pressure on the unpadded, bent elbow when the patient is lying supine) and brachial plexus palsy from over vigorous abduction in external rotation of the upper arm. Obviously pressure points should be adequately padded before committing a patient to general anaesthesia. A tourniquet or blood pressure cuff may also cause transient nerve damage. Weakness of the face has been known to occur from pressure on the facial nerve over the zygoma by the mask harness. Injection of local anaesthetic solution into any nerve may cause neuritis. Rarely, nerves are damaged from misplaced injection of irritant induction agents.

Epistaxis is common after nasal intubation. The use of a local vasoconstrictor before intubation will lessen its incidence. Packing the nasal cavity can control the haemorrhage afterwards. Epistaxis in younger patients is usually venous and easily controlled, but in older patients (60+) it may be arterial and difficult to stop.

Damage to the eye is fortunately rare. Corneal abrasions may be caused if the open eye is touched (the traditional attempt to elicit the corneal reflex during anaesthesia is not a good thing) or by the accidental spilling of irritants (including fluids used in skin preparation) into the eyes.

'Postoperative chests'

Factors which commonly precipitate postoperative chest lesions include:

1. The site of the operation (upper abdominal, and thoracic incisions limit coughing and deep breathing because of pain).
2. Pre-existing acute or chronic chest infections including chronic bronchitis which is often associated with smoking.
3. Pre-existing acute upper respiratory infections. Whatever the pressure placed on the anaesthetist by the operating team, patients scheduled for elective surgery should never be given a general anaesthetic if they are suffering from acute upper respiratory tract infections, such as common cold, sinusitis or sore throat.
4. Prolonged immobility during lengthy operations may prevent clearance of secretions.
5. The use of drying agents, and failure to humidify carrier gases in long procedures, may result in the sputum drying and becoming adherent, more viscous and difficult to clear by coughing. Humidification of the respiratory tract comes from within (from adequate intravenous hydration) as well as from without (humidification of anaesthetic carrier gases).

Chest lesions which may occur in the postoperative period include:

1. *Acute bronchitis.* This is common, and often pre-existing.
2. *Atelectasis.* This may be localised or massive. It results from obstruction of the bronchi by plugs of mucus which are not cleared by coughing or ciliary activity during general anaesthesia. Collapse of the lungs beyond the

obstruction results from absorption of the air. Collapsed lung easily becomes infected.

3. *Bronchopneumonia* is especially frequent in the elderly immobilised patient.

4. *Mendelson's syndrome* may occur after inhalation following gastric regurgitation or vomiting (Chapter 11).

The diagnosis and management of postoperative atelectasis. Pulmonary atelectasis should be suspected in any patient who, between 6 and 72 h after operation, has a temperature increased above 37°C with raised heart rate and a disproportionately increased respiratory rate. The diagnosis is confirmed by signs of patchy or widespread lung collapse on chest X-ray.

The diversity of attempted methods of management demonstrates that none is effective alone, but deep breathing, incentive spirometry and posture are used in many cases. If atelectasis is severe, transtracheal suction, intermittent positive pressure breathing and even bronchoscopy or reintubation may be necessary. Pain relief is important and may require the use of regional and peripheral nerve blocks.

Permanent brain damage

British courts take the view that far higher damages should be awarded to a patient whose brain is permanently damaged but survives than to those who die from anaesthetic or surgical mishap. This is because of the need to provide care for such tragic individuals.

If the heart stops from hypoxia, irreversible brain damage has probably already occurred (see also Chapter 14, Table 14.2). The signs include:

1. Fixed dilated pupils.
2. Failure to respond to surgical stimulation.
3. Persistent apnoea.
4. Loss or modification of electrocardiographic patterns (ECG).

Death

Death is the ultimate complication. It is often difficult to separate surgical pathology and the results of surgery from anaesthetic causes of perioperative death except when there has been an anaesthetic mishap. After all, no patient should have a general anaesthetic without a compelling surgical reason for it.

About one patient in 13,000–30,000 dies under or after general anaesthesia. The incidence varies from institution to institution, depending on the sort of surgery undertaken and the postoperative care available. A hospital which receives victims of major trauma is far more likely to record deaths on the operating table than a hospital caring for patients undergoing routine, elective surgery.

Anaesthesia can kill patients far too easily. The margin of safety if, for instance, the oxygen supply fails, is only 4–6 min before hypoxia results in permanent brain damage and 6–8 min before cardiac arrest supervenes. Nonetheless, the estimated mortality due solely to anaesthetic causes is now only about 1 in 180,000 anaesthetics.

14

Cardiopulmonary resuscitation

'. . . And Elisha lay down on the Shunamite child and
breathed life into him'
The Bible (Kings II, ll xxxii)

Resuscitation of the apparently dead by expired air respiration has been attempted over many centuries and is
mentioned in the Bible. Interest was renewed in the 17th
century, particularly in reviving the apparently dead after
drowning, leading to the invention of tracheal tubes, bellows
and other respiratory apparatus. There were also descriptions
of a variety of methods of supposed cardiac stimulation,
including blowing tobacco smoke up the anus. Methods of
artificial respiration such as those of Silvester based on
causing expansion of the chest by manipulating the arms and
compressing the chest, gradually became recognised as the
orthodox treatment of respiratory failure during the late nineteenth century[1]. Such methods held sway well into the 1950s
when expired air respiration (EAR) was reintroduced by the
Americans and Scandinavians.

---

[1] Was this partly because of the inate and hypocritical sense of
propriety developed in the Victorian era? One of the authors can
remember the outcry, even in the late 1960s in response to the the
suggestion that 'mouth to mouth' resuscitation should be taught to such
bodies as the Boy Scouts, student nurses and St Johns Ambulance Brigade
('All right for the continentals old boy, — but not for the British')

The aetiology of cardiac arrest

The expression 'cardiac arrest' implies that there is either absence of contraction (asystole), or the heart is beating so feebly or with such uncoordinated contractions that no blood is pumped round the circulation. Cardiac arrest can be primary (from disease or trauma, or due to cessation of the heart due to electrocution or drugs) or secondary (as the result of hypoxia following airway obstruction, centrally mediated respiratory arrest, or exsanguination).

Open cardiac compression via a thoracotomy or through the diaphragm from the abdominal cavity has been practised since the turn of this century, and direct (internal) defibrillation since the nineteen thirties, but it was the work of Kouwenthoven and his colleagues in the USA, published in 1960, which popularised external cardiac compression (ECC) and external electrical defibrillation, thus making resuscitation after cardiac arrest a more practical possibility[2].

Cardiac arrest in the operating suite, the intensive care or coronary care unit is a dreaded complication which may result from the inherent disease or condition of the patient; but it may also be precipitated by the procedures and drugs used in surgery, anaesthesia or treatment, due to unavoidable reflexes, side effects, mismanagement or accident. It is obvious that resuscitation is most likely to be successful in operating theatres, recovery rooms and other intensive care areas, where special expertise is available and equipment and drugs are to hand.

Respiratory arrest in the operating theatre is, as we have seen, commonplace and an elective part of many modern anaesthetic techniques. Central respiratory depression may be transient (after the administration of thiopentone for example) or due to elective peripheral paralysis by neuromuscular blocking

---

[2] The term 'cardiac *compression*' is more accurate and currently more favoured than the older expression 'cardiac *massage*'.

agents. The manoeuvres necessary to secure the airway by tracheal intubation anl instituting intermittent positive pressure ventilation (IPPV) by 'squeezing the bag', either manually or mechanically, are therefore second nature to anaesthetists[3].

Unanticipated loss of consciousness and/or respiratory and/or cardiac arrest outside the operating suite or intensive care area is a different matter and may occur inside the hospital in the general ward or outpatient department, or away from the hospital in a First Aid situation in a public place or in the home.

If sudden respiratory arrest or total obstruction of the airway occurs in a previously normally oxygenated patient breathing air, and the heart continues to beat effectively, there is probably between 6 and 8 minutes before the oxygen in the body is reduced to a level at which permanent damage to the brain develops. If primary cardiac arrest occurs and the circulation ceases immediately, there is at most five min before cerebral damage will be irretrievable. Every physician, nurse, medical student and all other paramedical personnel — and, indeed every intelligent member of the public — should know how to act if a patient suddenly becomes or is found unconscious (Fig. 14.1).

The ABC of the first aid 'basic life support' for the unconscious patient

The primary aim of the resuscitation of the unconscious patient is to ensure that the brain is oxygenated. This takes

---

[3] This was not always the case. Before the introduction of muscle relaxants in the 1940's respiratory arrest was regarded with dread second only to that afforded by a cardiac arrest. Its occurrence usually meant that anaesthesia had been carried too deep — to the point of apnoea. The surgeon had to stop operating, and artificial respiration was begun (often by chest compression methods rather than by IPPV).

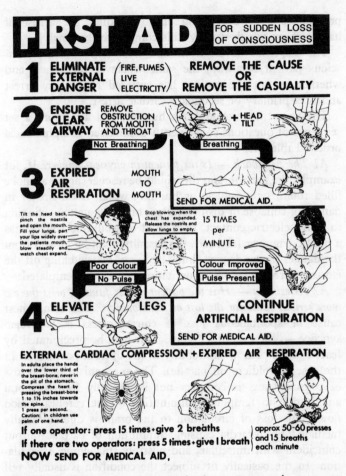

FIRST AID FOR SUDDEN LOSS OF CONSCIOUSNESS

1 ELIMINATE EXTERNAL DANGER (FIRE, FUMES LIVE ELECTRICITY) — REMOVE THE CAUSE OR REMOVE THE CASUALTY

2 ENSURE CLEAR AIRWAY — REMOVE OBSTRUCTION FROM MOUTH AND THROAT + HEAD TILT

Not Breathing | Breathing

3 EXPIRED AIR RESPIRATION — MOUTH TO MOUTH

SEND FOR MEDICAL AID.

Tilt the head back, pinch the nostrils and open the mouth. Fill your lungs, part your lips widely over the patients mouth, blow steadily and watch chest expand.

Stop blowing when the chest has expanded. Release the nostrils and allow lungs to empty.

15 TIMES per MINUTE

Poor Colour | No Pulse — Colour Improved | Pulse Present

4 ELEVATE LEGS | CONTINUE ARTIFICIAL RESPIRATION

SEND FOR MEDICAL AID.

EXTERNAL CARDIAC COMPRESSION + EXPIRED AIR RESPIRATION

In adults place the hands over the lower third of the breast-bone, never in the pit of the stomach. Compress the heart by pressing the breast-bone 1 to 1½ inches towards the spine. 1 press per second. Caution: in children use palm of one hand.

If one operator: press 15 times + give 2 breaths
If there are two operators: press 5 times + give 1 breath
NOW SEND FOR MEDICAL AID.

approx 50-60 presses and 15 breaths each minute

Fig. 14.1 Wall chart showing a scheme for the assessment and management without apparatus of a casualty who is found, or suddenly becomes unconscious. 'Mouth-to-mouth' expired air resuscitation (EAR) is shown as the method most usually taught but the authors and others believe that 'mouth-to-nose' EAR is an easier technique in many cases (see footnote, p. 235).

precedence over everything else (including the arrest of haemorrhage which usually kills comparatively slowly).

The sequence of diagnosis and treatment of the unconscious patient is always the same whatever the cause, and whether or not the patient has suffered respiratory arrest and/or a primary or secondary cardiac arrest.

The resuscitator should ask himself, and act upon, a set sequence of questions conveniently memorised in alphabetical order (Table 14.1).

A1 The Approach — Is the patient in physical danger? If, for example, the patient (and the would-be rescuer) are in a smoke filled room, or a vehicle or building which is on fire or in danger of collapse or disintegration, or the casualty is clinging to a live electric contact, or a child or would-be suicide has a plastic bag over his head, the casualty must be moved from the danger or the danger eliminated (e.g. by switching off the electric current) before resuscitation can be contemplated.

A2 Assessment — Has the patient merely fainted, or is there a more serious cause for the loss of consciousness? The commonest cause of spontaneous loss of consciousness is vasovagal syncope — the everyday 'faint'. This may be precipitated by fear, sudden pain or immobility in the upright posture (as in the case of soldiers on parade). The mechanism of the loss of consciousness is complex but is basically from cerebral anoxia due to temporary diminution of the cerebral blood flow. This loss of circulation to the brain is due to vagally mediated bradycardia causing diminution of cardiac output coincident with muscular, and possibly splanchnic, vasodilation. In the basically fit subject the condition is usually self limiting — the patient falls to the floor, the head is now below the level of the heart, blood rushes to the brain again, the patient regains consciousness and normal muscular and vascular tone is restored.

At the moment the patient falls to the floor he may be pulseless and intensely pale from constriction of the skin

Table 14.1 The first aid assessment and treatment of a patient who suddenly becomes or is found unconscious.

A.
1. The Approach
IS THE PATIENT IN PHYSICAL DANGER?
If 'Yes', either remove the danger or remove the patient from the danger
2. Asessment
HAS THE PATIENT MERELY FAINTED OR IS THERE A MORE
SERIOUS CAUSE FOR THE LOSS OF CONCIOUSNESS?
3. The Airway
IS THE AIRWAY OF THE PATIENT OBSTRUCTED?
If 'Yes', the obstruction must be removed and/or overcome by tilting the
head back and pushing the jaw forward or, in rare cases, bypassed.

B.
Breathing
IS THE PATIENT BREATHING?
1. If 'Yes', turn in to the lateral safe position and continue to hold the jaw forward.[1]
2. If 'No', institute expired air respiration (EAR) or manual or mechanical Intermittent positive pressure ventilation (IPPV).

C.
The Circulation
IS THE HEART CIRCULATING BLOOD TO THE BRAIN?
If 'No', external cardiac compression (ECC) must be started and EAR or
IPPV continued

D.
Definitive treatment.
If the heart recovers a coordinated beat spontaneously, consideration must
be given to the use of Drugs to sustain and improve cardiac output.
If the heart does not recover a coordinated beat spontaneously,
consideration should be given to determining whether any drugs should be
given prior to the use of . . . .

E.
Electricity
External defibrillation[2].

---

[1] If a spinal injury is suspected and the airway can be maintained by holding the jaw forward it may be wise to keep the patient supine to reduce the danger of possible damage to the spinal cord.
[2] In the case of an observed cardiac arrest with an external defibrillator immediately to hand (in a Coronary Care or Intensive Care Unit or in a mobile resuscitation ambulance) immediate defibrillation is often indicated before anoxia or acidosis develops.

vessels and may possibly be apnoeic. The appearance is not dissimilar to that of a primary cardiac arrest but it is obviously unnecessary and undesirable to begin EAR and ECC if the patient will recover spontaneously. The first acts of the resuscitator should, therefore, be to shake the patient gently, shout 'are you alright' and elevate the legs to increase the venous return to the heart. This takes less than 30 seconds but by then, if it is a simple faint, the colour will be coming back into the patient's face, respiration will be obvious, the pulse will be recovering in volume and rate, and the patient will begin to stir and open his eyes. The patient should then be turned into the lateral (recovery) position to avoid inhalation of gastric contents into the respiratory tree if he should vomit (see below). If the patient faints in the sitting posture his head should be thrust between his legs, usually with a similar satisfactory result.

A3 Is the airway obstructed? If the airway is obstructed oxygen (whether from air or an artificial source) cannot enter the lungs and be circulated to the brain in the blood stream, whether or not the patient is capable of making respiratory efforts, and whether or not the heart is contracting. The first objective must be to ensure that the airway is clear. Acute obstruction of the airway can be caused by:

1. The tongue falling back and obstructing the oropharynx and glottis.
2. Fluid or semi-solid material or foreign bodies obstructing the lumen of the upper air passages.
3. Compression from outside the air passages.

The relief of obstruction from the tongue falling to the back of the mouth is described in Chapter 6, Figure 6.1.

Fluid or semisolid material can be moved by sweeping the oropharynx with the fingers, preferably covered by a handkerchief or rag, and squeezing and wiping the nose (as a mother may do with her snotty-nosed offspring). The manoeuvres required to facilitate the expulsion of a solid foreign body or to bypass it if necessary were considered in Chapter 11.

Judicial hanging causes irretrievable damage to the spinal cord by fracturing the cervical vertebrae. Death from suicidal hanging is usually from asphyxia due to compression of the trachea and may be avoided if action is taken in time. The first act of the rescuer in such a case must therefore be to remove the ligature.

B1 Is the patient breathing? If there is no obstruction to the airway or the obstruction has been eliminated and the unconscious patient can draw air into the lungs, the immediate danger is over. All that remains is to turn the patient into the safe (semirecumbent) lateral position (Fig. 14.1). In this position the tongue falls forward and to the side, and vomited or regurgitated material will run out of the corner of the mouth. The patient must not be left unsupervised however, and it may still be necessary to push the jaw forward to keep the airway clear.

B2 If there is no obstruction to the patient's airway but the patient is not making respiratory efforts. Steps must be taken to fill the lungs with oxygen by inflation. In the first aid situation away from hospital this may mean that the only available methods are either 'mouth to mouth' or 'mouth to nose' expired air respiration (EAR). Expired air only contains 14% oxygen but this is considerably better than nothing. The rules are:-

1. Make sure the air passages are not obstructed and keep the jaw pushed forward.
2. Either close the nose by pinching it or close the mouth by tilting the head back and holding the jaw forward according to whether 'mouth to mouth' or 'mouth to nose' EAR is to be used.[4]
3. Spread your lips widely over the slightly open patient's mouth (or his nose) and blow steadily — watching out of the corner of your eye for chest expansion.

4. Lift your lips from the mouth or nose, separate the patient's lips slightly and allow full exhalation to take place.

C Is the heart circulating blood to the brain? If the patient is breathing spontaneously, the heart must be beating. If the patient's colour improves with EAR or mechanical IPPV, the heart must be beating. If the patient is not breathing and his colour does not improve with EAR or another form of IPPV (see below), and the major pulses (carotid or femoral) cannot be felt, the heart may either have arrested or be beating so feebly that the circulation is inadequate; external cardiac compression (ECC) is therefore indicated.[5]

External cardiac compression (ECC). Compression of the lower third of the sternum will squeeze the heart between the sternum and the vertebral column and raise intrathoracic pressure sufficiently to force blood round the arterial tree. The valvular system in the heart and compression of the venous system from the intermittently raised intrathoracic pressure allows only a forward flow of blood into the aorta. The heart will refill each time the pressure is relaxed provided that the patient is not dangerously exsanguinated.

[4] 'Mouth to mouth' EAR is most often taught but the authors and others believe that 'mouth to nose' is often easier and likely to be more effective, when no mechanical device such as a pocket mask or S-tube is available. This is because tilting the head back and pushing the jaw forward is the basic manouevre which opens a semirigid pathway through the nose and oropharynx to the glottis and respiratory tract (Figure 6.1). Depressing the jaw even slightly to part the lips for 'mouth to mouth' EAR tends to obstruct the oropharynx. 'Mouth to mouth' EAR may also be more difficult than 'mouth to nose' EAR if the patient has thickened or swollen lips.

[5] Confirmatory signs of cardiac arrest are: — absence of heart sounds when the ear or stethoscope is placed over the precordial area and dilation of the pupil. The latter sign is unreliable, especially if the patient has received medication, taken an intentional overdose or been poisoned. If the colour does not immediately improve with EAR or IPPV and the major pulses are absent, do not delay, begin ECC.

The recommended technique of ECC is:

1. Place the patient on a firm surface — the floor if necessary.
2. Locate the xiphisternum with two fingers.
3. Place the 'heel' of one hand just above these two fingers over the lowermost third of the sternum, and the other hand on top.
4. With the arms kept straight and rigid at the elbows, and moving from the shoulders, compress the sternum 4 to 5 cm (1 to 1½ inches) at a rate of 80 compressions/min (time each compression by saying 'one and, two and, three and, ... etc'). ECC is useless if the patient's lungs are not oxygenated. If the resuscitator is in the unfortunate position of being alone with the patient, he should pause every fifteen compressions to inflate the patient twice. If two resuscitators are present, the one administering ECC should pause every five compressions to allow a single inflation by the other.[6]

The signs of adequate basic life support for the patient who has sustained a cardiac arrest are:

1. Improvement in the colour of the patient.
2. A palpable femoral pulse and/or a carotid pulse with each compression of the chest.
3. Contraction of the pupils and opening of the eyes.
4. A struggling patient and signs of spontaneous respiratory effort as cerebral function returns.

If basic life support has been applied rapidly after cardiac arrest the heart may start to beat spontaneously, especially if the cardiac muscle is basically normal (e.g. after electrocution). The above signs of successful basic life support will then be present independent of ECC, although it may be

[6] It is difficult to learn EAR and ECC ('Basic life support') from a description or chart, and dangerous to practice on living volunteers or patients, but excellent manikins are available from Scandinavian firms such as Laerdal or AMBU International.

necessary to continue IPPV for a time if the patient is not breathing spontaneously.

If the above signs of adequate or reasonable cerebral perfusion are not present, ECC and IPPV are continued. Basic life support must be maintained until further measures (such as external electrical defibrillation) can be applied, either at the incident site or after the patient has been transported to hospital. Further definitive treatment of cardiac arrest which does not recover spontaneously (stage D in our alphabetical sequence) is discussed later in the chapter.

If, despite basic life support, the signs of adequate cerebral perfusion (improved colour, contracting pupil, respiratory effort, struggling, etc.,) are not present after a reasonable period of attempted resuscitation it will be necessary for the resuscitators or their leader to decide whether continuing is worthwhile. No arbitrary time limit can be set; the decision to declare the patient dead will depend on many factors including the geographical availability of drugs and apparatus for further treatment.

Aids to basic life support

Basic life support can be made more effective, and in the case of IPPV safer and more pleasant for the resuscitator, with the assistance of certain simple portable devices, some of which can be carried in a handbag or glove compartment of a car. It is surely reasonable to expect a medical practitioner to carry an emergency bag in the boot. It is, however, fundamental that the airway can usually be freed from obstruction, and EAR and ECC can be applied, without any mechanical aids whatever. Time is short, the would-be resuscitator must not hesitate to apply basic life support to the casualty in the absence of equipment, however distasteful a particular technique may be.

CARDIOPULMONARY RESUSCITATION 237

The airway can be more effectively cleared if an electric or foot operated sucker is available, and it can be more easily maintained if an oropharyngeal or nasopharyngeal airway is inserted to hold the tongue forward (Chapter 6), but obstruction can occur with a pharyngeal airway in place — the patient should always be turned into the safe position and supervised. Tracheal intubation (Fig. 14.2), now being taught to many paramedical as well as medical and nursing personnel, more effectively ensures a clear airway, particularly if the patient is to be transported, or ventilated with a self inflating resuscitation bag. Training and practice on models is essential as there is a real danger that the occasional intubator may pass the tube into the oesophagus.

The management of the totally obstructed upper airway was considered in Chapter 11.

Intermittent positive pressure respiration (IPPV) by EAR is not an aesthetic procedure. The recent development and spread of the HIV virus and autoimmune deficiency syndrome (AIDS) has increased apprehension amongst resuscitators. The HIV virus is of low infectivity; the spread of AIDS by EAR has never been recorded and there is doubt whether spread by saliva is possible. Nonetheless, the spread of other infections to the resuscitator is, at best, an unpleasant prospect. Those who are trained in EAR, and prepared to employ the technique, would do well to carry a portable device in the handbag, briefcase or pocket. Simple S-tubes and masks, which enable the resuscitator to blow into the patient's respiratory tree without contact with the lips have long been available (an ordinary anaesthetic mask is suitable). A further development is a valved device which directs the patient's expiration out of a different port or tube from that by the resuscitator. The latest version of the collapsible Laerdal® pocket mask is a well designed device which is especially useful with an oropharyngeal airway; the most

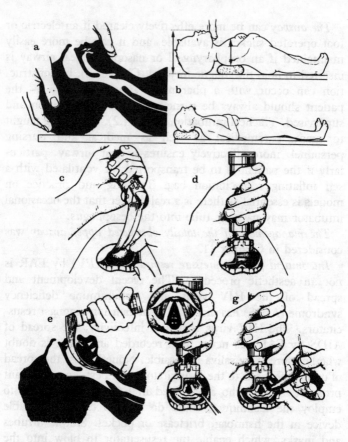

elaborate version has a nipple for adding supplementary oxygen (if it is available) to the resuscitator's expired air.[7]

Self-inflating resuscitator bags and one-way valves may be used for ventilating the patient with ambient air, which can

[7] Laerdal Medical Ltd, Goodmead Road, Orpington, Kent, BR6 OHX, England.

Fig. 14.2 Oral tracheal intubation: (a) The usual position for endotracheal intubation. The pillow is removed and the head is extended and the jaw held forward. (b) In children there is a proportionally larger anteroposterior diameter of the head; there will be too much flexion unless a pillow is placed under the shoulders. In older patients with kyphosis the pillow should be inserted under the occiput. (c) The lips are parted by the fingers of the right hand. The teeth are inspected. The Macintosh laryngoscope is inserted with the left hand from the right hand corner of the mouth, the tongue being packed away behind the guard on the left hand side of the mouth. (d) The epiglottis is visualised. (e) The tip of the Macintosh laryngoscope is inserted into the vallecula in front of the epiglottis. It is important not to 'lever' on the upper front incisors. The tongue and lower jaw should be 'lifted' with a steady pressure. (f) The larynx is exposed. The oesophagus is seen as a potential space posterior to the laryngeal opening. The cords may then be sprayed with local anaesthetic (4% lignocaine). The spray may then be passed between the cords to anaesthetise the trachea. (g) The endotracheal tube is inserted from the right hand corner of the mouth so that the bevel is correctly positioned and in order that the larynx may be kept in view until the last moment. A gentle 'conscious lift' should be given along the axis of the laryngoscope just before insertion to prevent 'drooping' the tip of the tube into the oesophagus.

The tracheal tube is shown without a cuff to make the illustration clearer. If the tube is cuffed the cuff should be blown up to just seal the trachea, a check made with a stethoscope to ensure that the tip is not in the right bronchus, and the tube then firmly secured by a bandage or adhesive tape.

Illustration drawn by Mr. Peter Cull, St. Bartholomew's Hospital, London. (Anaesthesia 1966. 21: 385).

---

be enriched with oxygen if it is available. The resuscitator bag may be connected to an anaesthetic mask (preferably with an oropharyngeal airway in place or a tracheal tube. There are many different models available; the original was the AMBU International bag with the Ruben valve.

Mechanical devices for the administration of closed chest cardiac compression have been described but they are not entirely satisfactory and they are not in general use.

The use of the electrical defibrillator is discussed later in this chapter.

Cardiac arrest in the operating suite

The causes of cardiac arrest in the operating suite include:-

The effect of drugs and/or disease on the patient

1. Dysrhythmias (usually ventricular fibrillation) either primary (e.g. due to myocardial or pulmonary infarction), hypoxia and/or certain drugs used in anaesthetic practice (e.g. adrenaline).
2. Hypotension due to hypovolaemia and/or drugs, such as relative overdose of some induction agents, (including thiopentone), certain muscle relaxants (e.g. tubocurarine) and local anaesthetics.
3. Allergic responses to certain agents (particularly some induction agents and muscle relaxants) which may precipitate the dangerous combinations of hypoxia due to bronchospasm and hypotension.

The effect of certain operative procedures.

1. Airway obstruction from tumours or laryngeal oedema.
2. Vagal stimulation from traction on viscera or intubation.
3. Sudden massive haemorrhage as may occur in major vascular or cardiac surgery.
4. Air embolism, as may occur in cardiac or neurological surgery.

Physical failure of technique or apparatus

1. Hypoxia from anatomical obstruction of the patient's airway or the kinking of an endotracheal tube, etc.
2. Hypoxia from failure of the oxygen supply (e.g. unnoticed emptying of cylinders, disconnexion or transposition of pipe-lines), or disconnexion of the patient from the apparatus (especially when a patient has been pharmacologically paralysed) or failure of a mechanical ventilator.
3. Electrocution due to faulty apparatus.

The diagnosis of cardiac arrest during general anaesthesia.

One of the most dangerous periods is during the induction of anaesthesia, but unfortunately, the degree of observation of monitoring devices may be minimal at that time, as the anaesthetist is concentrating on technical procedures such as intubation and manual inflation of the lungs. Venous access should be secured, and blood pressure apparatus, the electrocardiograph (ECG) and a pulse monitor (preferably a pulse-oximeter) should be applied before the start of the induction whenever possible. The absolute minimum requirement is for a trained assistant to be continuously palpating the pulse.

Cardiac arrest will be manifest during induction or maintenance of anaesthesia by cessation of respiration after a few gasps if the patient is breathing spontaneously, sudden deterioration in the patient's condition (including absence of the pulse by palpation or indicated on the pulse meter), failure to record blood pressure, pallor, cyanosis and a fall in saturation on the pulse oximeter, absence of capillary refill on compressing the face, and possibly by sudden dilation of the pupil.

A glance at the electrocardiograph will indicate whether circulatory arrest (asystole or ventricular fibrillation) has occurred or whether there is still a coordinated contraction and time to avert the impending catastrophe. It is essential to make sure that the ECG is properly connected; horror stories abound of drastic therapeutic measures being instituted when an apparent asystole resulted from the mere disconnexion of an ECG lead, or apparent ventricular fibrillation was diagnosed from an artifact on the trace — for instance, due to diathermy or the gain control mistakenly being set at maximum.

The ABC of immediate treatment of cardiac arrest during anaesthesia

1. Inform the surgeon and stop the operation — unless, of course, the cause of the arrest is an obvious sudden catastrophic haemorrhage.
2. Discontinue the anaesthetic.
3. Administer a precordial thump if the ECG indicates ventricular fibrillation or rapid ineffectual tachycardia. A precordial thump by the anaesthetist's fist may restore the situation by causing reversion to a coordinated rhythm. Repeated precordial thumps in complete heart block have been known to achieve an adequate cardiac output.
4. Initiate external cardiac massage and elevate the legs to increase venous return.
5. Make sure that you are able to administer oxygen from the apparatus by IPPV. Has there been a failure in oxygen supply or disconnexion of the apparatus from the airway? Is the endotracheal tube in the trachea? And if it is, is it free from obstruction? If it is obstructed, remove it. Has the unintubated patient vomited or otherwise obstructed? If there is doubt about the functioning of the apparatus use a manual self-inflating bag to ventilate the patient with air and added oxygen, or connect another anaesthetic machine, or, in the last resort, ventilate the patient by blowing intermittently down an endotracheal tube.
6. Replace blood volume rapidly with colloid or blood if hypovolaemia appears the primary or contributory cause of the arrest.

'D' The definitive treatment of cardiac arrest

If coordinated cardiac function (manifested by the continuance of the peripheral pulses when ECC is discontinued) does not return after basic life support, further treatment will be required. The heart may be in ventricular fibrillation or asystole. These may be distinguished on the ECG monitor.

Venticular fibrillation (VF) requires treatment by electric defibrillation. Modern defibrillators deliver a direct current (DC) shock of 80 to 400 joules. After charging the capacitators the electrodes are applied over broad areas below the right clavicle and below the left nipple.

If it is possible to deliver a defibrillating shock within 30 s of VF occurring — as may be the case in operating theatre or an intensive or coronary care unit — and/or basic life support (IPPV and ECC) was applied immediately after the arrest, metabolic acidosis may not have time to develop.

If more than one minute elapsed before basic life support was started, or IPPV and ECC have been continued for more than 5–10 min before an ECG and a defibrillator are available, sodium bicarbonate should be given (see (5) below) and IPPV and ECC continued for 30 s before electrical defibrillation is attempted.

The procedure is as follows:-
1. If the ECG shows ventricular fibrillation (VF) an immediate electric defibrillatory shock of 200 J should be administered from a DC (direct current) defibrillator[8].
2. If the VF persists and no peripheral pulse is palpable IPPV and ECC are continued for at least 15 compressions, and an increased shock of 400 J is administered. If this does not reverse the VF, another 400 J is given after further IPPV and 15 ECC compressions.
3. If VF persists 100 mg of lignocaine is adminstered intravenously as an antiarrhythmic, and another 400 J shock is applied after IPPV and 15 more ECC compressions.

[8] If a defibrillator is to hand, and a working ECG monitor is not available to distinguish between VF and asystole (in an ambulance for example), no harm will result if an electric defibrillatory shock is applied empirically.

4. If the VF remains resistant after this 4th shock, 10 ml of
   1 in 10 000 (a ten times dilution of injection of adrenaline
   BP) is given, and IPPV and ECC continued for 15
   compressions; after which another 400 J shock is
   administered.
5. If the VF still persists 50 ml of 8.4% bicarbonate should
   be administered before defibrillation is again attempted.

   Asystole is a more serious problem. Atropine may be given
intravenously while IPPV and ECC continue in an attempt
to restart the heart, but, if this fails, administer adrenaline
in an attempt to convert the heart to VF, and then proceed
with defibrillation.

Aftercare

The heart which has restarted after a cardiac arrest is in a
precarious state, but obviously those patients whose hearts
have suffered damage (as in myocardial infarction) are less
likely to survive than those whose cardiac arrest was due to
an acute episode such as electrocution or anoxia. Careful
titration of inotropic drugs (e.g. calcium, isoprenaline, dopa-
mine, etc.,) may be required, as well as antiarrhythmic drugs
such as lignocaine or beta-blockers, and electrical pacing of
the heart may be necessary.

   Other vital organs such as the brain and the kidney may
also have been damaged by hypoxia. Patients who have
survived cardiac arrests but have suffered irreversible neurological damage or complete brain death (Table 14.2) present
difficult and delicate social, legal and ethical problems which
may involve the decision to discontinue life support (mechanical ventilation, etc.,) and the possibility of donating trans-
plant organs.

Table 14.2 Criteria for establishing the diagnosis of brain death preparatory to the discontinuation of life support and possible organ donation.

The criteria and procedure outlined below are generally accepted by the medical and legal professions in the United Kingdom although a few practitioners still have reservations. It will be noted that the tests are primarily for 'brain stem' death and some residual abnormal electroencephalographic activity is not entirely excluded.

Preconditions
1. The diagnosis of brain death should not be made until at least 6 hours after the onset of coma or, in the case of coma following cardiac arrest, at least 24 hours after the restoration of the circulation.
2. The diagnosis of brain death must be made by two senior doctors (usually two consultants or a consultant and a Senior Registrar in the United Kingdom) either separately or together on at least two occasions with an interval of at least two hours between the examinations
3. There must be no doubt about the condition or circumstance which caused the coma.
4. Reversible causes for coma must be excluded; in particular depressant drug levels, the effect of muscle relaxants, hypothermia less than 35°C, and metabolic or endocrine disturbances.

Tests for the absence of brain-stem function.
The answer to *all* the following questions must be 'No':
1. Do the pupils react to light?
2. Are there any corneal reflexes?
3. Do the eyes move during or after caloric testing? This test involves first examining the ears to ascertain whether wax is present, and removing it if necessary, and then syringing the ear with ice cold water.
4. Are there any motor responses in the distribution of the cranial nerves in response to potentially painful stimuli of the face, limbs or trunk?
5. Is there a gag reflex if a catheter is introduced through the nose or mouth into the pharynx?
6. Is there a cough reflex if a catheter is introduced into the lower respiratory tract through the tracheal tube?
7. Is the patient completely apnoeic when the arterial carbon dioxide tension exceeds 7 kPa? An arterial sample must be taken and, if necessary carbon dioxide insufflated in to the respiratory tree by catheter until the $PaCO_2$ is brought up to the requisite level.

15

Epilogue: quality of anaesthesia

'The anaesthetist is a man apart, ... the patient's life is in his hands. The ease and perfection of an operation largely depend upon his skill . . . . The anaesthetist appears as a sort of prologue to the operation and then becomes an influence, pervading the whole action.'
The History of St. Bartholomew's Hospital, 1918.
Norman Moore, M. D.

The practice of anaesthesia is an unique combination of art and science. The patient is most affected by it but he is also the least likely to be aware of its successes or failures, since he is inevitably insensible at the time. Appreciation of the quality of the standard of care and the conduct of anaesthesia by the less discerning surgeon quite often depends only upon such crude criteria as whether the patient remained still or not during the procedure, whether he was sufficiently relaxed for abdominal surgery, or whether he was lucid afterwards and did not require an undue amount of postoperative care. The safety of the patient is the anaesthetist's prime responsibility. The quality of anaesthesia used to be measured by mortality, but now the death rate from anaesthesia is so low (probably one death in 180 000 anaesthetics in the United Kingdom) that it is a poor index[1]. Minor morbidity due to anaesthesia is often trivial compared to the pain or discomfort which surgery causes, but it is frequently magnified by the patient who can readily accept surgical complications but rarely expects problems related to anaesthesia. The well intentioned and, to some extent legally necessary, act of informing the patient in detail of the potential risks of anaesthesia may so frighten the patient that awareness of minor complications becomes more likely; a nice balance has to be struck at the preoperative visit by the anaesthetist.

The safety and comfort of the patient and the success of the anaesthetic rest squarely on the anaesthetist. The best anaesthetic is unnoticed by the surgeon and patient, and so the anaesthetist's only reward may be the self knowledge that he has done a good job.

This book has attempted to explain some of the responsibilities of anaesthetists and the methods used by them to come as close as possible to the goal of perfection. It only remains for the student to see these principles put into practice, and thus be enabled to form his own opinions about the specialty of anaesthesia.

---

[1] The overall mortality within 30 days of surgery from all causes (disease, surgery or anaesthesia) in over half a million operations studied in the United Kingdom by the *Confidential Enquiry into Perioperative Deaths (CEPOD)* was stated to be 0.7% in the report published in 1987.

Appendix A
Historical

'Today is yesterday's pupil'
Gnomologia 1732

Thomas Fuller, M. D.

BC

c. 2250   *Babylonian tablet* records
a dental filling of
henbane to relieve
toothache.

c. 500   *Hippocrates* described the
relief of pain by opium.

AD

c. 100   *Discorides* of Greece
administered a concoction
of the root of mandragora
to relieve the pain of
surgery.

c. 150   *Heron of Alexandria*
described the first
medical piston and barrel
syringe.

c. 250   *Hua T'o*, a Chinese
military surgeon, used
Indian hemp (hashish) to
render patients
unconscious for surgery.

c. 1200   *Nicolas of Salerno* gave an
account of the value of
inhalation of fumes from
the 'soporific sponge'
(soaked in hashish,
poppy (opium),
mandragora etc) for

surgical anaesthesia.
(Descriptions of the use
of the soporific sponge
persist throughout the
Middle Ages).

c. 1540   *Valerius Cordus*
synthesised 'sweet oil of
vitriol' and the Swiss
physician *Paracelsus*
described the induction
of sleep in chickens with
its vapour.

1596   *Sir Walter Raleigh*
(England) described the
effects of South American
native arrow poison —
possibly curare.

1665   *Sir Christopher Wren and
Sir Robert Boyle*
(England) observed the
effect of the intravenous
injection of opium into a
dog.

1730   *August Froberins*
(Germany) gave the name
'Ether' to sweet oil of
vitriol.

1751   *Bailey's English Dictionary*
defines anaesthesia as 'a
defect in sensation'.

248

1754 *Joseph Black* (Scotland) isolated carbon dioxide.

1766 *Franz Anton Mesmer* (Germany) publicised 'animal magnetism' (hypnosis).

1771 *Joseph Priestley* (England) discovered oxygen.

1772 *Joseph Priestley* (England) discovered nitrous oxide.

1794 *Thomas Beddoes* (England) founded the Pneumatic Institute at Bristol with the objective of treating chest diseases by the inhalation of gases and vapours.

1796 *James Moore* (England) produced local analgesia for the great John Hunter by compression of peripheral nerves.

1800 *Humphry Davy* (England) while acting as the superintendent of Beddoes Institute (see 1794) inhaled nitrous oxide thus reducing the pain of an erupting wisdom tooth. He suggested that the gas might be used for surgical anaesthesia.

1807 *Baron Larey* (France), Napoleon's great military surgeon, performed painless amputations on the frozen limbs of battle casualties.

1818 *Michael Faraday* (England) observed the analgesic effect of inhaling ether.

1824 *Henry Hill Hickman* (Ludlow, England) established the principle of 'suspended animation' (reversible surgical anaesthesia) by performing operations on animals under carbon dioxide anaesthesia.

1825 *Charles Waterton* (England) gave an account of the action of curare which he had brought back from South America.

1829 *Cloquet* (France) performed a mastectomy under hypnosis.

1842 *W. E. Clarke and Crawford W. Long* (both of the USA) independently made isolated use of inhaled ether for a dental extraction and the removal of a sebaceous cyst respectively.

1843 *John Elliotson* (England) published an account of his use of hypnosis for surgical 'anaesthesia'.

1844 *Horace Wells* (Hartford, Connecticut, USA) a dentist gave nitrous oxide to himself while his partner removed one of his teeth. He continued to use the gas successfully in his practise but failed at a public demonstration.

1844 *E. R. Smilie* (Boston, Massachusetts, USA) opened an abscess from a patient inhaling etheral tincture of opium from a sponge (the soporific sponge again!).

1846 *James Esdaile* (England) published details of his

use of hypnosis for surgery in India.

1846 *William Thomas Green Morton* (Boston, Massachusetts, USA) first administered ether for dental extractions in his own dental practice and then, on 16 October 1846, for the removal of a tumour of the neck at the Massachusetts General Hospital. Oliver Wendell-Holmes (Boston, USA)) attached the name 'anaesthesia' to Morton's discovery.

Dr. Francis Boott (an American living in London, England) received the news from Boston, USA and then persuaded the dentist *James Robinson* (London, England) to administer ether to a patient and extract a tooth under its influence on 19 December 1846. On the same day in Scotland an amputation was performed under ether at the Dumfries and Galloway Royal Infirmary, Scotland by *Dr. William Scott*. Scott had learned of the discovery from *Dr. Fraser* surgeon on the Cunard paddle steamer *Acadia* which had brought the news to England.

Robert Liston, the famous surgeon, performed the first 'capital' (major) surgical operation — an amputation — under ether in England on 21 December 1846 at the North London (now University College) Hospital. The anaesthetic was administered by a medical student William Squire.

1847 *James Robinson* (London, England — see 1846) published the first textbook in the world on anaesthesia — *A Treatise on the Inhalation of the Vapour of Ether*.

John Snow (London, England) becomes the first specialist anaesthetist and published his book — *On the Inhalation of Ether in Surgical Operations*.

James Young Simpson (Edinburgh, Scotland) introduced chloroform for the relief of pain in labour in November 1846.

1853 *John Snow* administered chloroform to Queen Victoria at the birth of Prince Leopold. This effectively silences theological doubts about the use of anaesthesia.

Alexander Wood (Edinburgh, Scotland) used a piston and barrel glass syringe and hollow needle to inject morphia subcutaneously in the vicinity of peripheral nerves to relieve neuralgia.

1857 *Claude Bernard* (France)

demonstrated that curare acts on the myoneural junction.

1858 *John Snow's book On Chloroform and other Anaesthetics* published posthumously.

1865 *Joseph Lister* (Glasgow, Scotland) introduced antiseptic surgery.

1870 *S. S. White* (USA) introduced liquid nitrous oxide cylinders.

1872 *Pierre-Cyprien Oré* (Bordeaux, France) gave intravenous anaesthesia with chloral hydrate.

1877 *Joseph T. Clover* (London, England) described his portable regulating ether inhaler.

1880 *William Macewen* (Glasgow, Scotland) introduced tracheal intubation for operations inside the mouth.

1884 *Carl Koller* (Vienna, Austria) introduced topical cocaine anaesthesia for ophthalmology.
W. S. Halsted (New York, USA) developed the use of cocaine by injection for local anaesthesia.

1885 *S. S. White* introduced compressed oxygen.

1887 *Frederic Hewitt* (London, England) described the first nitrous oxide and oxygen apparatus with cylinders.

1893 *F. W. Silk* (London, England) founded the London Society of Anaesthetists. The first such in the World and forebear of the Anaesthetics Section of the Royal Society of Medicine (1908), The Association of Anaesthetists of Great Britain and Ireland (1932), the Faculty of Anaesthetists of the Royal College of Surgeons of England (1948) and the College of Anaesthetists 1988.

1898 *August Bier* (Kiel, Germany) introduced clinical spinal anaesthesia.

1905 *The Long Island Society of Anaesthetists* was formed — forerunner of the *American Society of Anesthetists* (1913) and of *Anesthesiology* (1935).
Heinrich Braun (Germany) introduced procaine to clinical practice.

1912 *Arthur Läwen* (Germany) injected curare directly in to muscle to produce muscular relaxation for surgery.
James T. Gwathmey (New York, USA) produced his nitrous oxide, oxygen and ether apparatus.

1917 *Geoffrey Marshall* and *Edmund G. Boyle* (England) independently introduced machines for use by the British Army based on Gwathmey's.

1920 *Ivan W. Magill* and *E. Stanley Rowbotham* (London, England)

developed wide bore tracheal anaesthesia with nitrous oxide, oxygen and ether for use in plastic surgery.
Arthur E. Guedel (California, USA) published his first classic paper on the signs of anaesthesia.

1923 *Ralph M. Waters* (Winsconsin, USA) introduced carbon dioxide absorption.

1924 *P. Fredet* and *R. Perlis* (Paris, France) introduced somnifaine the first intravenous barbiturate anaesthetic.

1930 *Brian Sword* (Connecticut, USA) introduced the circle absorption system.

1933 *R. J. Minnitt* (Liverpool, England) promoted N_2O and air for obstetric analgesia.

1934 *Ralph M. Waters* (Winsconsin, USA) introduced cyclopropane.
J.S. Lundy (Minnesota, USA) introduced thiopentone.

1941 *C. Langton Hewer* (London, England) introduced trichloroethylene.

1942 *Harold R. Griffith* and *G. Enid Johnson* (Montreal, Canada) used intravenous curare with spontaneous ventilation in man.

1943 *R. R. Macintosh* (Oxford,

England) described his curved laryngoscope.

1946 *T. Cecil Gray* and *John Halton* (Liverpool, England) popularised the use of curare with controlled ventilation.

1947 *Torsten Gordh* (Stockholm, Sweden) introduced lignocaine.

1949 *Daniel Bovet* (France) introduced suxamethonium.

1956 *H. K. Beecher* (Boston, Massachusetts, USA) published his theories on pain.
Michael Johnstone (Manchester, England) and *Roger Bryce-Smith* (Oxford, England) introduced halothane.

1963 *L. J. Telivuo* (Sweden) introduced bupivacaine.

1965 *R. Melzack* (USA) and *P. D. Wall* (United Kingdom) described the gate theory of pain.

1966 *G. Corssen* and *E. F. Domino* (Michigan, USA) introduced ketamine.
R. W. Virtue (Colorado, USA) introduced enflurane.

1971 *A. B. Dobkin* (New York, USA) introduced isoflurane.

1977 *B. Kay* (England) and *G. Rolly* (Belgium) introduced propotol.

1984 *A. A. Spence and others* (Glasgow, Scotland) used propofol in a new formulation.

Appendix B
Further reading

'*Some books are to be tasted, others to be swallowed, and some few to be chewed over and digested*'
Of Studies.   Francis Bacon 1561–1626

For the medical student and the beginner.

Campbell D, Spence A A 1985 Norris and Campbell's Anaesthetics, Resuscitation and Intensive Care 6th edition. Churchill Livingstone, Edinburgh.

Evans T R 1986 The ABC of Resuscitation. British Medical Journal, London

Harrison M J, Healy T E J, Thornton J A 1984 Aids to Anaesthesia 1 and 2. Churchill Livingstone, Edinburgh

Lunn J N 1982 Lecture Notes on Anaesthetics, 2nd edition. Blackwell Scientific Publications, Oxford

Ponte J, Green W G Anaesthetics, Intensive Care and Pain Relief. Hodder and Stoughton, London

For the first year trainee and the occasional anaesthetist.

King M 1986 Primary Anaesthesia. Oxford University Press, Oxford

Smith G, Aitkenhead A R 1985 Textbook of Anaesthesia. Churchill Livingstone, Edinburgh

For reference.

Atkinson R S, Rushman G B, Lee J A 1987 A Synopsis of Anaesthesia, 10th edition. Wright, Bristol

Churchill-Davidson H C 1984 Wylie and Churchill-Davidson's A Practice of Anaesthesia, 5th edition. Lloyd-Luke (Medical Books), London

Historical

Átkinson R S, Boulton T B 1988 History of Anaesthesia. Royal Society of Medicine, London

Davison M H 1965 The Evolution of Anaesthesia. John Sherratt, Altrincham

Duncum B M 1947 The Development of Inhalation

Anaesthesia. Oxford University
Press, Oxford

Keys T E 1978 The History of
Surgical Anaesthesia. Robert E.
Krieger Publishing Company,
Huntington, New York

Rupreht J, Van Lieburg M J, Lee
J A, Erdmann W 1985
Anaesthesia. Essays on its history.
Springer-Verlag, Heidelberg

Sykes W S 1961, 1982 Essays on
the First Hundred Years of
Anaesthesia Volumes 1, 2 and 3.
Churchill Livingstone,
Edinburgh

Thomas K B 1975 The
Development of Anaesthetic
Apparatus. Blackwell Scientific
Publications, Oxford

Appendix C
Official British Pharmacopoeal (BP) and proprietary and other names

'What's in a name? That which we call a rose By any other name would smell as sweet'
Romeo and Juliet   William Shakespeare (1564–1616)

	Official BP Name	Proprietary Name
Analgesics	Morphine	Morphia
	Papaveritum	Omnopon
	Diamorphine	Heroin
	Pethidine	Demeral: Meperidine[1]
	Fentanyl	Sublimase
	Alfentanil	Rapifen
Anticlorinergics	Atropine	Atropine
	Hyoscine	Scopolamine
	Glycopyrrolate	Robinul
Sedative phenothiazines	Chlorpromazine	Largactil: Thorazine
	Promethazine	Phenergan
	Trimeprazine	Vallergan
Benzodiazepines	Diazepam	Valium: Diazemuls
	Nitrazepam	Mogadon
	Flurazepam	Dalmane
	Lorazepam	Ativan
	Temazepam	Euhypnos: Normison
	Midazolam	Hypnovel
Intravenous anaesthetics	Thiopentone	Pentothal: Intravel: Thiopental[1]

[1] United States Pharmacopea.

255

	Official BP Name	Proprietary Name
	Methohexitone	Brietal: Brevital: Methohexital[1]
	Etomidate	Hypnomidate
	Propofol (di-isopropyl phenol)	Diprivan
	Ketamine	Ketalar: Ketaject
Inhalation anaesthetics	Nitrous oxide	'Gas' (colloquial)
	Cyclopropane	'Cyclo' (colloquial)
	Ether (di-ethyl ether)	Letheon (historical)
	Trichloroethylene	Trilene: Trimar
	Halothane	Fluothane
	Enflurane	Ethrane: Alyrane
	Isoflurane	Forane: Herrane
Muscle relaxants	Tubocurarine	'Curare' (colloquial): Tubarine
	Gallamine	Flaxedil
	Alcuronium	Alloferin
	Pancuronium	Pavulon
	Atracurium	Tracrium
	Vecuronium	Norcuron
	Suxamethonium	Scoline: Anectine
Anticholinesterases	Neostigmine	Prostigmine
	Edophonium	Tensilon
Phenothiazine anti-emetics	Perphenazine	Fentazin
	Prochlorperazine	Stemetil
Other anti-emetics	Metoclopramide	Maxolon, Primperan
	Droperidol	Droleptan
	Cyclizine	Valoid
Antidotes etc.	Naloxone (opioids)	Narcan
	Doxapram (central depressants)	Dopram
	Flumazenil (benzodiazepines)	Anexate

Index